For Emma,

Xmas 2000

Love,

Alan + Diana

DEMOCRACY

and

DNA

DEMOCRACY

and

DNA

AMERICAN DREAMS AND
MEDICAL PROGRESS

GERALD WEISSMANN

HILL AND WANG

NEW YORK

Library of Congress Cataloging-in-Publication Data
Weissmann, Gerald.
Democracy and DNA : American dreams and medical progress / Gerald
Weissmann.
p.   cm.
Includes bibliographical references and index.
1. Medicine—United States—History—19th century. 2. Medicine—
United States—History—20th century. 3. Progress.
4. Humanitarianism. 5. Medical innovations—Social aspects—United
States. 6. United States—Civilization—19th century. 7. United
States—Civilization—20th century.   I. Title.
R152.W46 1996   610'.973—dc20   95–46250   CIP

For Ann,
who introduced me to
much of what this book is about: America

CONTENTS

I do not know that I should feel threatened or insulted if a chemist should take his protoplasm or mix his hydrogen, oxygen, and carbon, and make an animalcule incontestably swimming and jumping before my eyes. I should only feel that it indicated that the day had arrived when the human race might be trusted with a new degree of power, and its immense responsibility; for these steps [are] only a hint of an advanced frontier supported by an advancing race behind it.

—Ralph Waldo Emerson, 1871

. . . the growing good of the world is partly dependent on unhistoric arts, and that things are not so ill with you and me as they might have been is half owing to the number who lived faithfully a hidden life and rest in unvisited tombs.

—George Eliot, 1872

A term for which I am indebted to George Eliot [is] meliorism. By this I would understand the faith which affirms not merely our power of lessening evil—this nobody questions—but also our ability to increase the amount of positive good.

—James Sully, 1877

. . . though I admit to a sanguine temperament, I prefer to describe myself as a "meliorist"—one who believes that the world can be improved by finding out what is wrong with it and then taking steps to put it right.

—Sir Peter Medawar, 1984

INTRODUCTION

If poverty is an evil, or disease a misfortune, then certainly, where they coexist, the miseries of each are intensified by the presence of the other, and the sum total is multiplied an hundred fold . . . it follows that society must still continue to provide for those of its members who are, by either of these calamities, incapacitated from taking care of themselves.

—H. G. Clark, *Outlines of a Plan for a Free City Hospital*, Boston, 1860

No city in history has professed more ardently the belief that social reform is the sister of medical progress than Boston before the Civil War, which Dr. Oliver Wendell Holmes called the Hub and Van Wyck Brooks called the city of Dr. Oliver Wendell Holmes. Boston was the hub not only of the American Renaissance but also of a broad social movement in the Western democracies that came to be called meliorism. Meliorism differs from simple altruism by virtue of its belief in progress through reason rather than sentiment. An altruist feeds the beggar; a meliorist feeds the beggar and vaccinates his children. Meliorism, I believe, is the spirit that unites the age of abolition with the age of DNA, American dreams with medical progress, and in this book I will use chapters from the lives of nineteenth-century abolitionists and reformers, many of them eminent Bostonians, as a framework for the claim that modern molecular biology is perhaps the most lasting expression of the meliorist spirit. And since those who presided over the Flowering of New England would have been pleased by the Flowering of DNA, the meliorist voice of Dr. Holmes will be heard frequently. It should not be difficult to recognize *The Autocrat of the Breakfast Table* as a model for the narrative structure of this book.

When James Russell Lowell was offered the editorship of a new literary magazine in 1853, he had made it "a condition precedent" that his friend Dr. Oliver Wendell Holmes be the first contributor engaged. Holmes had at the time a reputation chiefly as the author of "Old Ironsides," as a lyceum lecturer, and as Boston's most brilliant conversationalist. But he accepted Lowell's challenge of steady work and published his feuilletons in every issue of the new journal. He also gave the publication its name. *The Atlantic Monthly* may be said to be Holmes's godchild. (We are still in debt to his knack for names. Holmes not only christened Boston the Hub but also coined the term anesthesia; in his novel *Elsie Venner* he introduced "Brahmin" as the label for Boston's finest class.) In addition, he imported the study of medical microscopy from France to the United States, demonstrated the cause of childbed fever, and invented the parlor stereopticon. A short, feisty gamecock of a man, dedicated to medical education and reform, he was, for a time, dean of the Harvard Medical School. As an unabashed sanitary crusader, Dr. Holmes was proud to be a member of the skeptical medical community of Boston, which today—as in 1869 when he addressed it—holds "every point of human belief, every institution in human hands, and every word written in a human dialect, open to free discussion, today, tomorrow, and to the end of time."

It was a book of his essays, *The Autocrat of the Breakfast Table*, that made the literary reputation of Dr. Oliver Wendell Holmes. Those humorous pieces, unstructured products of a magpie mind, were transcripts of the doctor's thoughts "dipped from the running stream of consciousness"—the phrase made famous by his student William James. In twelve volumes of verse and prose, Holmes raised the flags of wit and reason against provincial, sentimental, and politically pious people, whom he called "moral bullies." As the conflict grew between North and South, as sanitarian joined abolitionist and Brahmin closed ranks with Free-Soiler, his wit turned blunt and his tone sharp. In the glum days after his son was wounded at Ball's Bluff he wrote to his friend John Lothrop Motley in England:

> I have a most solid and robust faith in the [cause of the] North, in its endurance, its capacity for a military training, its plasticity for every need, in education, in political equality, in respect for man as man in peaceful development, which is our law, in distinction from aggressive colonization; in human qualities as against bestial and diabolical ones; in the Lord as against the Devil. If I never see peace and freedom in this land, I shall have faith that my children will see it. If they do not live long enough to see it, I believe their children will.

Abolitionist and sanitarian alike believed that the Union's defense of "human qualities as against bestial" fulfilled the Puritan charge to do God's work on earth. But the men and women of reform had become impatient with the doctrinal disputes of their stern Puritan fathers and expected to be judged by deed, not creed—a nineteenth-century belief that became the motto of the Ethical Culture movement. Many of us believe that perhaps the most splendid deed of the late twentieth century has been the Flowering of DNA, and this book will trace this great biological revolution to its roots in meliorist soil. Aspects of the meliorist tradition have been passed to us from Dr. Holmes to Lewis Thomas, from Margaret Fuller to Albert Szent-Györgyi, from Thomas Wentworth Higginson to James Watson, and from Katharine Lee Bates to David Baltimore.

Meliorism may also be defined as the social mission of the liberal imagination. Its adherents believed that rational thought applied to human actions would change the social order to increase the sum of pleasure over pain. George Eliot tells us in *Middlemarch* that medical science is the jewel in the crown of meliorism, because it forms a "direct alliance between intellectual conquest and social good." It was probably no accident that she coined the term "meliorism" in 1876 after a generation of medical and social reform had changed the face of Victorian England. And it is in the service of sanitary reform that Tertius Lydgate and Dorothea Casaubon join to build the fever hospital in Middlemarch. Eliot's fictional Lydgate studies medicine in the Paris hospitals that taught the real Oliver Wendell Holmes; Lydgate also served as one model for the hero of Sinclair Lewis's *Arrowsmith*, a book now unread by those whose idea of a doctor is a "health care provider." Alas, not only the rise but the fall of heroic medicine and of meliorism have coincided.

These days, meliorism seems out of favor; it has become synonymous with shallow optimism. Its scientific and literary bases are both under siege. In the trendy news pages of *Nature*, the historian W. F. Bynum claims that "the historical reverberations of AIDS [are] a salient reminder that meliorism is a hollow philosophy in 1994." From the sterner columns of *The New Criterion*, Roger Kimball dismisses C. P. Snow and one half of *The Two Cultures*: "in the end, Snow is a naive meliorist. For him . . . science is the means of raising the standard of living, ergo science is the arbiter of value." And from the heights of the bestseller list, E. L. Doctorow, on behalf of his hero in the novella *The Waterworks*, dismisses the "trinomial" stars of the American Renaissance—Thomas Wentworth Higginson, James Russell Lowell, Dr. Oliver Wendell Holmes, and Henry Wadsworth Longfellow: "Their names were too long for the work they produced."

We might ask Bynum and his friends of the left whether anything *except* meliorist science will help stanch the reverberations of AIDS; we might ask Kimball and his friends of the right what arbiter would value *not* raising the standard of living of ordinary people. As for Doctorow, one might argue that Higginson's

Army Life in a Black Regiment, Lowell's "Commemoration Ode," Holmes's "The Chambered Nautilus," and Longfellow's "The Psalm of Life" need no apology.

Other critics of meliorism aim directly at its scientific base. Since science is expressed in words that vary with time and place, they argue that science is *only* an expression of that given time and place. In academic jargon, since science is only one form of socially determined *discourse* and since the *text* of science is contingent on its *context*, science cannot be value-free. That notion is not novel. Addressing his fellow members of the Massachusetts Medical Society in 1857, Dr. Holmes made the same point, *sans* jargon, pointing out the very close relation between "the Medical Sciences and the conditions of Society and the general thought of the time. . . ."

Medicine and science have not been permitted to follow their independent paths in every time and place; changes of "the conditions of Society and the general thought of the time" have made the road a rocky one. Earlier in our century, the notion that there is no such thing as value-free science—or medicine, for that matter—was mainly championed by National Socialists or Stalinists of the Lysenko school. But nowadays, fifty years after the purges of "Jewish physics" and "capitalist genetics," the social-construct camp has attracted a crop of more well-intentioned devotees. Liberal proponents of feminism and diversity, and a majority of new historians, philosophers, and sociologists of science, believe that science, by definition, is the construct of those who do it. They also believe that science has been mainly pursued in the interest of those who pay for it, an establishment of white, male Europeans. There is no such thing as a scientific truth, they tell us, only a temporary construct that society permits to be true. Western, "objective" science is simply coercion in optimist clothing. This argument derives from academic analyses of the social sciences and the arts, and may have some merit in those fields. The text of a work of art, Congreve's *Way of the World*, for example, is indeed studied gainfully in the context of Restoration comedy. But a scientific text of the period, Boyle's statement of the behavior of ideal gases, or $pV = nRT$, is clearly independent of its origin in Restoration science. That's the difference between a perfect play and a perfect gas.

Well, the lions of academe have long been as liable as the rest of us to ignore evidence that shatters their dearest belief. At the height of the McCarthy era, when liberals and left-wing activists were menaced and purged all over America, Lionel Trilling taught in an English Department that was high on the Henrys, both Adams and James, that debated the political "ideas" of Yeats, Eliot, and Pound, and that cherished contemporary Southern "nativists" such as Allen Tate and John Crowe Ransom, yet he believed: "In the United States at this time liberalism is not only the dominant, but even the sole intellectual tradition."

In the chapters that follow I will suggest that the scientific, if not always the literary, culture of our time has remained true to Trilling's belief in the liberal imagination. Indeed, it might be argued that our modern, reductive approach to the human genome and its manipulation is an extension of the meliorist passion to understand and to heal, of the meliorist urge to examine the body politic by what George Eliot called the "serene light of science." We shall see, for example, how the long campaign for women's rights in the United States, which Margaret Fuller launched in 1849, came to owe as much to abolitionists and sanitarians as to the Transcendentalists of Brook Farm. Those Yankee movements, those American dreams, left behind them not only a rich literature and the politics of social justice, but also clean water, urban health, child labor laws, and the settlement-house movement. Their legacy includes New York's Central Park, Boston's Mount Auburn Cemetery, and two great American anthems of social justice (Julia Ward Howe's "Battle Hymn of the Republic" and Katharine Lee Bates's "America the Beautiful").

It should not surprise us that among the first sanitarians was Dr. Samuel Gridley Howe—Julia's husband—who named their home Green Peace and who devoted his life equally to social causes and to the study of blindness. Referring to his front-line work in the Greek war of independence, Holmes called him "the Grecian and blind-compelling Dr. Howe." An abolitionist to the core, Howe protested at an 1846 rally the return of a fugitive slave to Louisiana: "The port of Boston has been opened to the slave-trader; for God's sake, Mr. Chairman, let us keep Faneuil Hall free! Let us devise such means and measures as shall secure to every man who seeks refuge in our borders all the liberties and all the rights which the law allows him." Dr. Howe was only one of many nineteenth-century reformers in whom sanitarian and meliorist urges were combined. In our own century, the messy divorce between those who aim for intellectual conquest and those who work for social good has been painful to watch.

But the Flowering of New England was no unspoiled garden of reason and light. The purely literary masters of the period, Hawthorne, Melville, and Thoreau, not to speak of Emerson in his "Brahma" mode, had different American dreams, believing as they did that the Yankee concern for material progress would lead to spiritual impoverishment. Hawthorne looked back with nostalgia to the golden age of *The Marble Faun* to complain, "The entire system of Man's affairs as at present established makes us all parts of a complicated scheme of progress, which can only result in our arrival at a colder and drearier region than we were born in . . . We go all wrong, by too strenuous a resolution to go all right." Many transcendentalists were great fans of Thomas Carlyle and his cult of the hero. Believing in the principle of "emotive intellection," they were convinced that reform began with the inner self. But their humorless pursuit of the tragic led them to Swedenborg and Mesmer, and the clotted notions of irrational thinkers like these have come around again. These days Thoreau's different drummer wears the motley of

MTV and leads armies of herbalists, crystal freaks, homeopaths, and spiritualists who march under the banner of what Sir Peter Medawar has called Pluto's Republic. "A specter haunts our culture—it is that people will eventually be unable to say 'They fell in love and married,' let alone understand *Romeo and Juliet.*" So Trilling worried in 1950; he was afraid that Freudian jargon would garble the narrative art. Half a century later the specter that haunts our culture is not Freud, not Marx, but Godzilla. And that was Romeo who?

As we stagger to the finish of this anxious millennium, scores of the mindless announce a New Era, but the New Age they await is the Age of Unreason. Ancient rituals and outworn prattle are displacing sweetness and light. The marketplace of ideas has become a souk of attitudes. Another of George Eliot's admonitions is apt here: "The notion that what is true and, in general, good for mankind is stupid and drug-like, is not a safe theoretic basis in circumstances of temptation and difficulty."

As a social mission, meliorism seemed to have run aground at mid-century, perhaps because it had no answer to Auschwitz. But, as the motive for medical progress, meliorism is very much afloat, precisely because the atrocities and horrors of the death camps were so clearly devoid of meaning. The meliorist tradition of Western science has always been based on two complementary notions. The first is that the need to know is wired in our genes and demands unfettered inquiry, a playful hunt for facts. (Aristotle: "all men by nature desire to know.") The second is that useful meaning can be plucked from the thicket of fact. Therefore, meliorists do not accept the distinction commonly made between "basic" and "applied" science. They believe that there is only applied science and science which has not yet been applied.

The last sentence of the paper by James Watson and Francis Crick which announced the double helix may be said to have begun the Flowering of DNA: "it has not escaped our notice that the specific pairing [of bases in DNA] we have postulated immediately suggests a possible copying mechanism for the genetic material." That paper, unlike two others that accompanied it in the same issue of *Nature*, by Maurice Wilkins and Rosamond Franklin, is immortal not because of the data, its facts, but because of its unique attention to base-pairing as an element common to the structure *and* function of DNA, its application. The two other papers make no reference to a copying mechanism, and it is the single conjecture of function, wrought from the many facts of DNA structure, that gives the Watson-Crick paper its overriding éclat.

Mark Twain once quipped that "there is something fascinating about science. One gets such wholesale returns of conjecture out of such a trifling investment of fact." The obverse was true of the Flowering of DNA. Before Watson and Crick, scientists had harvested wholesale returns of facts aplenty: "transforming principles," "purine and pyrimidine structures," "base ratios," "hydrogen bonding"; these wanted only the "trivial investment" of a genial guess, a mechanism. The chemistry and physics of DNA turn out to obey laws as universal as those of Boyle's perfect gas. But just as $pV = nRT$ describes the behavior of gases in a rocket to the moon or a mortar in Sarajevo, the ratio of G:C and A:T are equal in the DNA of finch and earthworm, mouse and microbe, tanager and Trilling. The clock that sets the time to copy DNA was figured out in quahogs; the truth of our new biology is that we are such stuff as clams are made of.

It would be reassuring for many of us were the truths of medical science simply a collection of tall stories we could take or leave at will—texts of comfort or terror, of promise or warning, but tales after all of the mind, texts without bite. Marianne Moore described the world of poetry as composed of imaginary gardens with real toads in them. Well, I'm afraid that the truths of medical science are those of *real* gardens with real toads in them. They are not the baubles of one race, one gender, one class, or one Reich. They have been worked out by the buzzing of eager minds despite the nattering complaints of the pious, the zealous, the mystic, and the inspired. The ultimate law of our science is, after all, its method. Science cannot guarantee life, liberty, or the pursuit of happiness—it is only a way of solving problems, a kind of constraint on the imagination, on the tall story and humbug. Those who share the meliorist dream believe that we can use our science to keep us free; if we're lucky, we can have Democracy and DNA.

I. ANTEBELLUM BRAHMINS

O beautiful for patriot dream
That sees beyond the years
Thine alabaster cities gleam
Undimm'd by human tears!
America! America!
God shed his grace on thee
And crown thy good with brotherhood
From sea to shining sea!

—Katharine Lee Bates, "America the Beautiful," 1893

1. KATHARINE LEE BATES RETURNS FROM PIKE'S PEAK

"Sweet land"
at last!
out of the sea—
the Venusremembering wavelets
rippling with laughter—
freedom
for the daffodils! . . .

Einstein, tall as a violet
in the lattice-arbor corner
is tall as
A blossomy peartree.

—William Carlos Williams, "St. Francis Einstein of the Daffodils,"
on the first visit of Albert Einstein to the
United States in the spring of 1921

Katharine Lee Bates (1859–1929) is the most famous native of Falmouth, Massachusetts; her statue decorates the library lawn, the road to the library bears her name, the bicycle path along Vineyard Sound to Woods Hole is named "The Shining Sea," and the upscale granola store is called "Amber Waves." Naturally. When Falmouth celebrated the centenary of her verses, about fifteen hundred listeners spread themselves on the large green lawn before the town library on a lovely August afternoon. Some had brought folding chairs and picnic baskets; children and dogs romped about. The crowd was composed of townsfolk and tourists, summer residents and day-trippers; there was a smattering of scientists and staff from the nearby Woods Hole Oceanographic Institution and the Marine Biological Laboratory. The uniform was summer dress: baseball caps and straw bonnets, pedal pushers and khaki shorts, madras and Keds. Sunburns.

An enormous American flag (courtesy of Atkinson Plumbing and Heating) covered most of the stone facade of the library annex. Wooden trestles had been set up before it to hold the performers. The Epic Brass quintet, imported from Boston, warmed up the crowd with a virtuoso display of tuba and trombones. Finally the chorus formed itself in tiers before the flag; the 100-member, amateur Greater Falmouth Mostly All-Male Men's Chorus (including twenty-nine women singing tenor parts and one woman baritone) wore red, white, and blue tennis shirts and uniformly friendly grins. Conducted by Thomas Goux, choir director of Falmouth's First Congregationalist Church, of which Bates's father had been minister, the chorus proceeded to take the audience on a "musical tour of America from sea to shining sea." The tour included the "Navy Hymn," for Falmouth is an oceangoing town, "Shenandoah," "Home in Sweet Missouri," "The Cowboy Lullaby," "Colorado Trail," and "My Sweet Wyoming Home." The selections were received with happy applause; the chorus did not disappoint its many well-wishers. "BREAK A LEG!" urged the Falmouth Orthopedic Associates in the program. The first part of the program ended with a sentimental rendition of Emma Lazarus's poem that decorates the Statue of Liberty, "Give Me Your Tired, Your Poor . . . ," with music by Irving Berlin.

The Epic Brass provided suitably patriotic toots and parade sounds for the ice-cream-and-soft-drink break, and when the chorus reassembled for the second half of the concert, we were treated to "America the Beautiful" in the most familiar setting (by Samuel A. Ward):

O beautiful for spacious skies
For amber waves of grain,
For purple mountain majesties
Above the fruited plain!
America! America!
God shed his grace on thee
And crown thy good with brotherhood
From sea to shining sea!

During that first verse, for which chorus and crowd joined together a cappella, I remembered Williams's poem about Einstein. In the middle of that corny Norman Rockwell pageant of small-town Americana, the image presented itself to me of Liberty raising her beacon hand beside the golden door to "Einstein . . . tall as a blossomy peartree." It struck me that the American notion of "brotherhood from sea to shining sea" had made it possible for Einstein—and other refugees from Hitler's Reich, including my parents—to settle here permanently. Some of those refugees became the grandfathers of DNA: Max Delbrück, Erwin Chargaff, Salvador Luria. Were it not for that sentiment of brotherhood, some of us would not have been sitting cheek by jowl with Yankees at the town library of Falmouth, Massachusetts. It's a sentiment less bellicose than that expressed in our official national anthem and considerably sweeter than the boast of "Deutschland über Alles," the pomp of "God Save the Queen" or the gore of "La Marseillaise." It was a fine song for a group of Americans to be singing in the sunshine and I turned to the program of the concert to find out more about Katharine Lee Bates.

Bates got the idea for "America the Beautiful" on her first trip out West. A professor of English at Wellesley, she had been asked to teach English religious drama at a summer school in Colorado Springs, where she happily spent "three weeks or so under the purple range of the Rockies." To celebrate the end of the session, she and others on the faculty made an excursion to

Pike's Peak, pulled to the summit by mules in prairie wagons that bore the slogan "Pike's Peak or Bust!"

"It was at the summit, as I was looking out over that sea-like expanse of fertile country spreading away so far under those ample skies, that the opening lines of the hymn floated into my mind," she wrote.

She left Colorado Springs with notes for the entire four stanzas and other memorabilia of her extended trip to the Rockies, but the poem did not appear until July 4, 1895, in *The Congregationalist*. After a musical setting by the once well-known Silas G. Pratt attracted national attention, the popular stanzas became open game for other musical versions, and by 1923 more than sixty "original" settings had been perpetrated. The verses can be sung to many old tunes including "Auld Lang Syne" and "The Harp That Once Through Tara's Halls." But the setting we know best nowadays was adopted by Samuel Ward from the hymn "Materna" and the words we use are those of Bates's revised version of 1904.

In Falmouth, we listened to the second stanza sung to the stirring music of Clarence G. Hamilton, the Wellesley organist of Bates's time, for it was her favorite setting:

> O beautiful for pilgrim feet,
> Whose stern, impassioned stress
> A thoroughfare for freedom beat
> Across the wilderness!
> America! America!
> God mend thine ev'ry flaw,
> Confirm thy soul in self-control
> Thy liberty in law!

Those lines could serve as a motto for Bates and her impassioned generation of Pilgrim daughters. Bates was graduated from Wellesley in 1880, ten years after that stern seminary-style college had been chartered as a place for "noble, white unselfish

Christian Womanhood." But by 1882 winds of change from the West brought a new generation. Alice Freeman (1855–1902) was only twenty-seven years old when she was called from the co-educational University of Michigan to become Wellesley's second president. She proceeded to transform the seminary into a college ready for the twentieth century. Among her first appointments were Eliza Mosher as professor of practical physiology and Katharine Coman (also from Michigan) as professor of political economy and history. In 1885, she appointed Katharine Lee Bates an instructor of English. In 1897, they were joined by Mary Calkins—a student of William James—who established the first laboratory of experimental psychology to be headed by a woman. Like Mosher, Coman, and Calkins, Katharine Lee Bates was destined to spend her entire, unmarried life at Wellesley; she became full professor in 1891 and long-term chairman of the English Department until her retirement in 1925. "I think she carried the idealism she had for individuals to the department itself," wrote her colleague Vida Scudder. "It was to her always the 'dear department.' " The qualities attributed to Alice Freeman were shared by her associates, women who "combined an extraordinary degree of intensity of feeling with absolute self-control." Indeed, "Confirm thy soul in self-control" could be said to have been the guiding principle of the plucky women who established scholarship at Wellesley.

I looked around at some in that audience at Falmouth who wore college T-shirts from Radcliffe, Harvard, MIT, Vassar, and the Marine Biological Laboratory. These men and women were institutional heirs of those pioneering women. Alice Freeman, as president of Boston's Woman's Education Association, collaborated with Elizabeth Cary Agassiz (widow of the biologist) to work out the legal arrangements whereby the Harvard Annex for women attained institutional standing as Radcliffe College. The Woman's Education Association also raised $10,000 to promote the teaching and research of women in science, a gift that made it possible in 1888 to purchase land near the all-male U.S.

Fisheries building at Wood's Holl (as it was then) to establish
the Marine Biological Laboratory. The WEA also insured that
women might work at the laboratory by requiring the presence
of two of its members on the board of trustees: the first two
were graduates of Vassar and MIT.

In 1893, the year of her trip to the West, Katharine Lee Bates
and her travel companion, Katharine Coman, stopped at the
great Columbian Exposition in Chicago. By that time Alice
Freeman had become Alice Freeman Palmer, having married a
Harvard philosopher, and the Palmers had supervised construction and installation of the Woman's Building on the fairground.
This upbeat monument shone in alabaster among the Beaux Arts
structures of "The White City" in the Exposition. The alabaster
city gleamed, indeed!

The Woman's Building was not the only reason why Katharine Lee Bates "was naturally impressed by the symbolic
beauty of the White City." She and Katharine Coman had
taught in Colorado Springs on equal terms with Professors Rolfe
of Harvard (Shakespeare) and Todd of Amherst (astronomy);
Coman had lectured on the economic history of Western expansion; and it was at the Chicago fair that Frederick Jackson
Turner delivered his famous address, "The Role of the Frontier
in American History." He argued that the Western frontier had
for three centuries been a metaphor for the American dream,
for "manifest destiny"; now that the open frontier had closed
and the United States had become one nation from ocean to
ocean, other frontiers awaited. Coman's two-volume *Economic
Beginnings of the Far West* was devoted to parallel themes, and
her economic history of the railroads again echoed Turner's
message that the age of an external frontier and the West as
wilderness was over. Coman and Bates were convinced in 1893
that the spirit that had won the West would in time breach the
internal frontier of inequality. America's "ev'ry flaw" would
yield to the stern, impassioned stress of reform: "thy liberty in
law."

The third stanza, perhaps the weakest poetically, was sung to the martial beat of John Carroll Randolf's Sousa-like measures:

> O *beautiful for heroes proved*
> *In liberating strife,*
> *Who more than self*
> *their country loved*
> *And mercy more than life!*
> *America! America!*
> *May God thy gold refine,*
> *Til all success be nobleness*
> *And ev'ry gain divine!*

The America of continental expansion was no collection of White Cities. The year 1893 was one of significant social unrest, and the strife was by no means liberating. Grover Cleveland entered the White House for the second time with the country in the midst of a deep economic depression. On February 23, 1893, the Philadelphia and Reading Railroad had gone bankrupt and before the end of the year the Erie, the Northern Pacific, the Union Pacific, and the Atchison, Topeka and Santa Fe went belly-up as well. Two and a half million people were unemployed—one fifth of the workforce—and Henry Adams lamented that "much that had made life pleasant between 1870 and 1890 perished in the ruin." Even the President admitted that "values supposed to be fixed are fast becoming conjectural, and loss and failure have invaded every branch of business." In legislation that was to provide windfall profits for J. P. Morgan and for August Belmont, Cleveland brought the country back to the gold standard in the very week that Bates stood atop Pike's Peak.

Meanwhile, federal and state militias were sent against workers in the Carnegie (Homestead) steel strike, against switchmen in Buffalo and coal miners in Tennessee, and finally into the Pullman strike in Chicago the next year. Each of these episodes of class warfare was later treated in Katharine Coman's *Industrial History of the United States* (1905). The record of American troops in those campaigns did not persuade Bates and Coman that our heroes loved "mercy more than life." The crisis of the 1890s probably explains Bates's hope that God—and not J. P. Morgan—might refine the nation's gold. Doggerel or not, "Til all success be nobleness" sounded a stern, antimaterialist tone that would have made the Pilgrims proud.

The second stanza of William Carlos Williams's "St. Francis Einstein" begins:

> *O Samos, Samos*
> *dead and buried. Lesbia*
> *a black cat in the freshturned*
> *garden. All dead.*
> *All flesh they sung*
> *is rotten . . .*

Katharine Lee Bates and Katharine Coman lived together for more than a quarter of a century in the cozy bonds of what then was called a "Boston marriage." Their Wellesley home they called the Scarab, their faithful collie Sigurd, and their automobile Abraham (because they were so often deep in its bosom). Bates as a person combined great human warmth and humor with a stern sense of values. A student reported that "her unwieldy body and slow movements were in Falstaffian contrast with her agile, almost legendary wit." Vida Scudder remembered Coman as "somewhat awe-inspiring, but alluring," and the two women were both productive scholars and devoted teachers. "I ought to be a live coal in their midst," wrote Bates of her students, "and they ought every one to catch fire."

They were also in the vanguard of social activists. Bates and Coman were among the founders in 1887 of the College Settlements Association, a group that made it possible for young women college graduates to spend a year at community settlement houses among the poor and the immigrants—the "teeming refuse" of Europe's shores. In the course of this work they became closely associated with the pioneer of Chicago's Hull House—and future Nobel Peace Prize winner—Jane Addams. In 1889, Addams's lifelong companion, Ellen Gates Starr, described how the settlement-house movement might benefit not only the needy but also the philanthropist: "It is not the Christian spirit to go among these people as if you were bringing them a great boon: one gets as much as one gives [but] people are coming to the conclusion that if anything is to be done towards tearing down these walls . . . between classes that are making anarchists and strikers the order of the day, it must be done by actual contact and done voluntarily from the top." A generation of social workers, public-health activists, and egalitarians spent their lives convinced of the need for "actual contact."

In 1892, Katharine Coman became chairman of the committee that opened Denison House in Boston; she made it a center of labor-organizing activity to which Bates was inevitably drawn. Denison House, Hull House, and the other settlement houses were deeply committed to reform of working hours, protection of immigrants, compulsory school attendance, school health, and—above all—abolition of child labor. It was toward this end that the poet Sarah Cleghorn wrote in *The Masses*:

> *The golf links lie so near the mill,*
> *That almost every day,*
> *The laboring children can look out*
> *And see the men at play.*

When violence broke out during the Chicago Pullman strike of 1894, and strikers burned down the remnants of the White City, Coman and Addams sided with workers against the militia; Coman went to Chicago again in 1910 to help striking seamstresses win union rights. Coman's last major work, com-

pleted as she lay dying of cancer, was a study of how other
countries cared for the aged, the disabled, and the unemployed,
Unemployment Insurance: A Summary of European Systems.
The book's call for old-age and disability benefits in the United
States—social security—became a platform plank of the Progressive and then the Democratic parties. After the New Deal,
Coman's dream became the law of the land. Bates describes
how she helped her friend finish this major work of social analysis:

> *Through those four years beset with wasting pain,*
> *The surgeon's knife again and yet again,*
> *. . . So we twain*
> *Finished your book beneath Death's very frown.*
> *For all the hospital punctilio,*
> *Through the drear night within your mind would grow*
>
> *Those sentences my morning pen would spring*
> *To meet . . .*

Those lines come from a volume of passionate love poems,
Yellow Clover, written by Bates and published in 1922, seven
years after Coman died. Each of these poems is devoted to
Katharine Coman and in some Bates reached levels of emotional
expression—perhaps even art—that eluded her in seven other
volumes of verse.

> *Your life was of my life the warp and woof*
> *Whereon most precious friendships, disciplines,*
> *Passions embroider rich designs . . .*
>
> *No more than memory, love's afterglow?*
> *Our quarter century of joy, can it*
> *Be all? The lilting hours like birds would flit*
> *By us, who loitered in the portico*
> *Of love's high palace . . .*

Bates spoke in no loud voice the love that dared not speak its name: yellow clover stood for physical love in the flower language of the two Wellesley scholars, who

> *Stooped for the blossoms closest to our feet*
> *And gave them as a token*
> *Each to each*
> *In lieu of speech,*
> *In lieu of words too grievous to be spoken,*
> *Those little, gypsie wondering blossoms met*
> *With a strange dew of tears? . . .*

"Freedom for the daffodils!" cried Dr. Williams decades later. Freedom for yellow clover! he might have urged. Nothing buried in the American garden, ever again! we would hope. "Undimm'd by human tears" sounded the hopeful lyrics of Bates's most successful public poem, our national anthem of social justice, a hymn to the better angels of American nature. The lyrics remain a memento of two noble lives, Coman's no less than Bates's, and a living monument to a generation of women whose reforms outlasted the alabaster cities' gleam of the Columbian Exposition. That generation of Americans made it possible for all of us in Falmouth that afternoon—men and women, straight and gay, black and white, town and gown—to sing peacefully together on the sunlit green lawn of the library the wonderful last verse of "America the Beautiful":

> *O beautiful for patriot dream*
> *That sees beyond the years*
> *Thine alabaster cities gleam*
> *Undimm'd by human tears!*
> *America! America!*
> *God shed his grace on thee*
> *And crown thy good with brotherhood*
> *From sea to shining sea!*

2. DR. HOLMES RETURNS
FROM PARIS

In 1833 Oliver Wendell Holmes wrote to his parents in Boston, "I am more and more attached every day to the study of my profession, and more and more determined to do what I can to give my own country one citizen among others who has profited somewhat by the advantages offered him in Europe." He had taken the road that many other ambitious young men from the provinces had taken; he was in Paris to study medicine and for the young American the experience was more bracing than even a Yankee spring:

> I am getting more and more a Frenchman . . . I love to talk French, to eat French, to drink French every now and then (these wines are superb, and nobody gets drunk, except as an experiment in physiology); and I do believe, if Napoleon was alive, and I stayed here much longer, I should want to fight a little . . . I have become attached to the study of truth by habits formed in severe and sometimes painful circumstance and self-denial. For, trust me, the difficulties in the investigations of our profession, the carelessness and stupidity—often the obstinacy—of patients, the cold and damp and loathsomeness of the dissecting-room, are exceedingly repulsive to the beginner.

But he persevered, and brought the gift of the new observational medicine back with him to Boston. He was also a factor

in connecting the trinomial men of the American Enlightenment
with the scientific spirit of Paris.

> The more I see of French character, the more I am delighted
> with it. I have hardly heard an— As I was writing this,
> [Ralph] Waldo Emerson came up to see me. He had been
> sitting some time when I heard another knock, and in
> walked—James Russell [Lowell]! I never was so astonished
> in my life; but as he is here, and I must attend to him, without
> ceremony I shall take the liberty to conclude my letter . . .
> Give my love to everybody.

The so-called Flowering of New England followed upon the
commercial success of Boston after the American Revolution,
and similarly, a medical revolution followed the intellectual success of Paris after the Revolution and the Napoleonic years.
Boston and Paris were very different cities in the 1830s, but both
had outgrown the rigors of their *anciens régimes*, and reform
was in the air, medical no less than social. Holmes looked back
at that time in both cities to argue:

> Medicine, professedly founded on observation, is as sensitive
> to outside influences, political, religious, philosophical, imag-
> inative, as is the barometer to the changes of atmospheric den-
> sity. Theoretically it ought to go on its own straightforward
> inductive path, without regard to changes of government or
> to fluctuations of public opinion. But [there is] a closer rela-
> tion between the Medical Sciences and the conditions of So-
> ciety and the general thought of the time, than would at first
> be suspected.

The notion that experimental medicine and social reform have
common origins in the "atmospheric density" of Paris in the
1830s was also suggested in two very different works of imaginative literature, George Eliot's *Middlemarch* and Edgar Allan

Poe's *The Murders in the Rue Morgue*. Poe's book of 1841—
the first murder mystery—has an epigraph that comes from
one of Holmes's favorite writers, Sir Thomas Browne, the
seventeenth-century Oxford-trained physician and author of the
classic *Religio Medici*: "What song the Syrens sang, or what
name Achilles assumed when he hid himself among women, although puzzling questions, are not beyond *all* conjecture."
Browne might therefore be called the ancestor of the murder
mystery, for proposing that even the most puzzling questions
might yield to conjecture.

Poe, however, properly gets full marks for having invented
the genre and for showing us that when the game's afoot the
corpses don't stay in their urns. In the *Rue Morgue*, which is
set in Paris of the 1830s, one of them is found up the chimney.
Poe's detective, the Chevalier Auguste Dupin, identifies the
murderer, who turns out to be not a human but an ape, which
he knows about from "a generally descriptive account of the
large fulvous Ourang-Outang of the East Indian Islands" in
Baron Cuvier's treatise of zoology. Dupin clinches his case by
finding at the crime scene "this tuft of tawny hair, [which] is
identical with that of the beast of Cuvier." Dupin might be said
to have caught his murderer by means of the latest genetic tech-
niques of the day. The hint of DNA in fiber evidence, so to
speak.

The ubiquitous Baron Georges Cuvier (1769–1832) pretty
much founded the science of comparative anatomy, and there is
Poe's ape, on pages 87 and 88 of the first volume of the Baron's
five-volume contribution to deforestation, *Le Règne Animal*.
Poe got the beast just right; not bad for a West Pointer! Clearly,
Poe's detective must have studied both nature and books very
closely, since his solution of the murders in the *Rue Morgue*
depended not only on the hair of the beast but also on Cuvier's
description in minuscule 8-point type.

Poe filled his work with more accounts of dissection, galvanic
experiments, wasting diseases, and near-death experiences than

one might find in the current books on the best-seller list of *The New York Times*. While his stories are called "tales of terror and the imagination," they can also be read as case histories of death and dying. Written in the shop talk of his decade's pathology, they tend to yield a whiff of the morgue. Marie Roget's autopsy, for example, with its "bleeding cellular tissue," or M. Valdemar's "left lung, which had been for eighteen months in a semi-osseous or cartilaginous state," could—and may have—come from G. L. Bayle's textbook *Recherches sur la Phthisie Pulmonaire* (1815). And in his role as narrator, Poe often describes clinical methods favored by the most advanced practitioners of his day. In "The Gold Bug," the narrator asks Poe's hero, Le Grand, why he is so deeply affected by a secret cipher:

> "My dear Le Grand," I cried, interrupting him, "you are certainly unwell, and had better use some little precautions. You shall go to bed, and I will remain with you a few days, until you get over this. You are feverish and . . ."
>
> "Feel my pulse," said he.
>
> I felt it and, to say the truth, found not the slightest indication of fever.
>
> "But you may be ill and yet have no fever. Allow me this once to prescribe for you . . . And will you promise me, upon your honor, that when this freak of yours is over, and the bug business (Good God!) settled to your satisfaction, you will then return home and follow my advice implicitly, as that of your physician?"

It was during Poe's lifetime that medicine started on its path to being an exact science from its source in pastoral art, and Paris was the setting. The key step in that transformation was the introduction of clinimetrics, the numerical recording of a patient's vital signs (pulse, temperature, and respiration). It was unusual, before the nineteenth century, for doctors to record their findings quantitatively. A clinical revolution followed hard upon this metric revolution, and both were wrought in the City of Light. After pulse and temperature were recorded routinely, doctors could begin to settle their puzzling cases not by "conjecture" but by comparing them with other cases compiled in books. Those compilations became useful when vital signs had been reduced to precise numbers and when statistical methods could be applied to the course of disease. The *cause* of disease, on the other hand—its pathologic anatomy—was sought at the dissecting table or in the morgue, where dead bodies were brought for identification. On the rue Morgue, victims of murder, suicide, or accident became the stuff of medical knowledge. Charles Méryon's chilling etching shows the quayside mortuary ready to receive the night's cargo from scows on the river. Since the bodies were sold for cash to students of medicine and art alike, it could be said that surgery and realism came of age by the Seine.

For the day-to-day story of medical life in 1830 Paris we need not turn to Poe or George Eliot, however. No account of that macabre traffic rings truer than that of the twenty-four-year-old Oliver Wendell Holmes. He had arrived in Paris for clinical training after his student days at Harvard and was thrilled by the opportunity:

The whole walls around the École de Médecine are covered with notices of lectures, the greater part of them gratuitous; the dissecting-rooms, which accommodate six hundred students, are open; the lessons are ringing aloud through all the great hospitals. The students from all lands are gathered together, and the great harvest of the year is open to all of us . . .

It is an odd thing for anybody but a medical student to think of, that human flesh should be sold like beef or mutton. But at twelve o'clock every day, the hour of distribution of subjects, you might have seen Bizot and myself—like the old gentlemen one sometimes sees at a market—choosing our day's provision with the same epicurean nicety. We paid fifty sous apiece for our subject, and before evening we had cut him into inch pieces. Now all this can hardly be done anywhere in the world but at Paris [where anyone] who gives his attention exclusively to the subject for a time, may, as I have said I have done, become an expert operator in a few weeks. I have told you all this to let you know that I am not staying at Paris for nothing.

As Holmes was writing this, Paris was filled with American, English, German, and Austrian medical students. They were drawn to the one city in the world where, thanks to an abundance of hospitals and a new spirit, clinical medicine was becoming an observational science. And perhaps the greatest attraction of the École de Médecine was Professor Charles P. A. Louis. A generation of young American doctors traveled to Paris to walk with him on the wards and to study his books. He was an early proponent of clinimetrics and drilled his students to record the pulse, the temperature, and the respiration. Louis was also the founder of clinical research in France; his work on what we would call patient outcomes led to the abandonment of bloodletting or leeches as treatments for infection. He began the Society of Clinical Observation, to which Holmes was admitted and the principles of which Holmes brought back to America. Holmes wrote to his parents in 1834:

Everything is now perfectly favorable to my progress in my studies. I am master enough of the language to take a case from a patient, write it off, read it uncorrected, and defend it against criticism, in a society of Frenchmen. There will be no difficulty in my obtaining any advantages I may desire here. My belonging to the society I have mentioned brings me into contact with young men in [good posts in] most of the hospitals, lays their experience before me, and puts me under the obligation to be exact, methodical, and rigorous. Besides, as I told you before, I have undisputed entrance at all times to two wards, containing together a hundred beds, generally full, where I examine and pound and overhaul the patients before even Louis or his interne have seen them.

To the end of his life, Holmes would remember the mantra of Louis, the proverb of scientific medicine:

> *Formez toujours les idées nettes.*
> *Fuyez toujours le à peu près.*
>
> *(Formulate your ideas precisely.*
> *Always avoid the approximate.)*

The large central hospitals of Paris were a legacy of the Revolution and of Napoleon; the new scientific spirit was a legacy of a young genius named Xavier Bichat (1771–1802). Bichat's theory that disease resides not in organs, but in tissues, conquered Europe and was brought to American shores by doctors from Boston, Philadelphia, and New York. Years later, Holmes asked:

> And is it to be looked at as a mere accidental coincidence, that while Napoleon was modernizing the political world, Bichat was revolutionizing the science of life and the art that is based upon it; that while the young general was scaling the Alps, the young surgeon was climbing the steeper summits of unexplored nature; that the same year read the announcement of those admirable "Researches on Life and Death," and the bulletins of the battle of Marengo?

After Bichat, the ambition of the School of Paris was to describe tissues and their ailments at the grand, systematic level of a Lamarck or a Cuvier. Medicine was to become as encyclopedic in its descriptions as paleontology or zoology: *Formez toujours les idées nettes.* But more: because doctors could now measure vital signs quantitatively, they could decide whether their treatments were helping or hurting their patients. Louis's great contribution was a statistical study that clearly showed bloodletting (phlebotomy) to be useless in the treatment of febrile diseases. Holmes's praise was just: "I consider his modest and brief 'Essay on Bleeding in Some Inflammatory Diseases,' based on cases carefully observed and numerically analyzed, one of the most important written contributions to practical medicine, to the treatment of internal disease of this century."

Bichat and Louis changed the way that doctors spoke to each other about patients and disease. Before the School of Paris, case records were history at best, anecdote at worst, but conjecture always. After Bichat and Louis, causality and numbers took over the medical record: *Fuyez toujours le à peu près*. And since clinimetrics taught doctors that the poor died earlier and more brutally than gentlefolk, scientific medicine became an aspect of social reform. Meliorism was born at the bedside.

George Eliot's fictional Tertius Lydgate goes to Paris in 1829 because there is "scientific work to be done which might have seemed to be a direct sequence to Bichat's." Lydgate sets out to find the "primitive tissue," spending tedious days with scalpel and microscope and devoting long nights to galvanic experiments. The microscope comes back with him to Middlemarch, where he has visions of launching into clinical research à la Louis. But then he meets Rosamond Vincy and settles for fine furniture instead of medical reform. Lydgate, on the verge of marrying Rosamond, takes one last glance at his fervid youth:

> his more pressing business was to look into Louis' new book on fever, which he was especially interested in because he had known Louis in Paris and had followed many anatomical demonstrations in order to ascertain the specific differences between typhus and typhoid. He went home and read far into the smallest hour, bringing a much more testing vision of details and relations into this pathological study than he had

ever thought it necessary to apply to the complexities of love and marriage.

The new spirit of the École de Médecine in the 1830s, the "testing vision of details and relations," is captured by Holmes in a letter which explains to his friend John Sargent why he cannot write poems for *The New England Magazine*, recently bought by Sargent and "the Grecian and blind-compelling" Dr. Samuel Gridley Howe:

> I am at the present moment living not merely the most laborious, but by far the most unvaried and in its outward circumstances most unexciting mode of life that I have ever lived. Nearly five hours in the day I pass at the bedside of patients, and you may imagine that this is no trifling occupation, when I tell you that it is always with my notebook in my hand; that I often devote nearly two hours to investigating a difficult case, in order that no element *can* escape me, and that I have always a hundred patients under my eye. Add to this the details and laborious examination of all the organs of the body in such cases as are fatal—the demands of a Society of which I am a member—which in the course of two months has called on me for memoirs to the extent of thirty thick-set pages—all French, and almost all facts hewn out one by one from the quarry—and my out-of-door occupations have borne their testimony . . . No, John, a heavier burden from my own science, if you will, but not another hair from the locks of Poesy, or it will be indeed an ass's back that is broken.

Holmes's youthful letters from Paris predict the qualities he was to show in his medical and literary careers: ambition, energy, and wit, qualities which he placed in the service of "intellectual conquest and social good"—George Eliot's phrase for the medical urge. Similarities between the letters of young Holmes, unpublished in Eliot's lifetime, and the musings of

Lydgate reflect not only common meliorist aims but the sense of hope and excitement that followed the clinical revolution of the School of Paris. Incidentally, they make Michel Foucault's revisionist story of those years, *The Birth of the Clinic: An Archeology of Medical Perception* (1973), seem slightly shabby. Paris in the 1830s was a mecca of science and medicine that lives as much in fiction as in fact. In that Paris of the mind, a young Tertius Lydgate will drop forever his galvanic experiments to finish his evening studying the oeuvre of Bichat or Louis. Poe's Auguste Dupin will snoop forever around the morgue while Oliver Wendell Holmes shops for bodies at fifty sous a pop. Louis Agassiz is in the cellars of the Jardin des Plantes drawing fish scales and ape bones for Baron Cuvier's atlas. Bayle's students by candlelight will study forever the tissues of Marie Roget. And poor Edgar will die in the hospital of drink and tuberculosis, with lungs turned to cartilage like M. Valdemar's. The illustrations are etchings by Charles Méryon with blackbirds aplenty.

The Paris of 1830 was also the time and place of Honoré de Balzac. It has therefore not escaped literary critics that the city was midwife not only to the murder mystery but also to the realistic novel. "Is it to be looked at as a mere accidental coincidence," to use Holmes's phrase, that it was also the time and place where modern medicine was born? The mystery's search for Whodunit (the murderer) and the doctor's search for Whatdunit (the microbe) share a common vocabulary. The clinical and criminal investigator both launch an inquiry, follow a protocol, unravel the evidence, and find a solution at the end. The realistic novel—which one might call a search for Whohasit and Whogetsit—surrenders its solution at the very beginning: character.

Were *Middlemarch* to have been written as a murder mystery the victim would have been Tertius Lydgate, young man of science. Whodunit? The most obvious suspect would have been charming Rosamond, who diverted her husband from science to the fireside. But *Middlemarch* is a Victorian novel, and therefore from our earliest meeting with the young doctor we already know that Tertius himself will be the culprit. His character dictates his choice. He will—because he must—become Tertius Lydgate, an uxorious doctor who treats the affluent for gout. We are not surprised: Eliot has already told us that in his Paris days "it was to be feared that neither biology nor schemes of reform would lift him above the vulgarity of feeling that there would be an incompatibility in his furniture not being the best." This statement of character is a very English way of rephrasing Prudhomme: "I'd rather die for the common man than live with him for a week." There is a precedent in Stendhal's *The Life of Henri Brulard*: "I would do anything for the happiness of the people, but I would rather, I think, pass a fortnight out of every month in prison than live with those who dwell in the shops." Lydgate shares this fondness for ease and the comfort of class; Eliot and Stendhal present us with two characters whose nature determines that reform will have to wait a while.

What the gene is to the cell, character is to the Victorian novel: a code of instruction that dictates the plot. In our own time, the instructions for molecular biology have been written by bookish people. After we've cloned our *libraries* of genomic DNA, as they put it, we look for the *open reading frames* of one or another genes; we ask if they have been *faithfully transcribed* and *correctly translated*; soon the human genome will be an open text awaiting deconstruction. One might say that the genres of medicine seem to be following certain genres of literature. In step with the literary fashions of *their* day, the observational medicine of the nineteenth century flourished as the novel came of age, and the systematic medicine of the eighteenth century had followed the path of the *Encyclopedia*. Zeitgeist is as zeitgeist does.

Medical historians tell us that nineteenth-century doctors were not the first to extract clinical teaching from the case histories of single patients. Indeed, the liberating concept that teachers of medicine could distill the name of one illness from stories of many is an end product of Enlightenment medicine. It is to d'Alembert and Diderot that we owe our capacity to clump and classify disease. The *philosophes*, by practice and example, taught doctors how to trim the tree of medical knowledge—to borrow a phrase from Robert Darnton. Indeed, before doctors could recognize clinical syndromes (literally: that which goes together) they had to have seen many sick patients in one place at more or less the same time. That happened in England during the early industrial revolution when the rural poor were herded into London workshops south of the Thames. In Paris, the *sans-culottes* were stuck in warrens east of the Bastille. Doctors at Guy's Hospital in London or St. Antoine in Paris could now see in a week more cases of one disease than their predecessors had encountered in a lifetime. Instead of *patients*, doctors now saw *cases* gathered in factorylike hospitals. And so was born nosology. Nosology—the simple classification of diseases —achieved maturity in the century between the founding of Guy's Hospital in 1734 and the revolution in clinical observation launched by Louis at the Hôpital la Pitié. That introduction of clinical observation changed medicine once and for all—much in the way that the realistic novel changed literature once and for all. And Dr. Holmes brought back to the United States the medical if not the fictional news from Paris.

In 1834 Dr. Holmes brought Louis's model for a society of clinical observation home to Boston, and by introducing microscopy to the Harvard Medical School shortly thereafter he laid the foundation for what were to become the Clinical-Pathological Conferences of *The New England Journal of Medicine*. It was by means of Louis's quantitative methods—the same methods that had discredited bloodletting—that Holmes was able to determine that puerperal fever, a childbirth fever that we now know is caused by streptococcal infection, was carried to and from infected women by doctors, nurses, or midwives.

One reason that few nineteenth-century women entered American hospitals to give birth was that before doctors learned about microbes, as many patients died from hospital infection as were helped by being bedded down. Not only "poor Edgar"—Holmes's phrase for Poe—died in the hospital. And even in the course of home visits doctors, midwives, and nurses seemed likely to spread infections. Holmes figured this out with respect to childbirth fever in 1843, years before the Hungarian clinician Ignaz Semmelweis made the same observation in Europe. Holmes, like the detective who was to be named for him, was able to deduce the pattern of transmission of puerperal fever by carefully examining the case records of the condition in New England.

Holmes personally contacted doctors in whose practices puerperal sepsis seemed to cluster. One doctor wrote to Holmes about a "disastrous period in my practice": between July 1 and August 13, 1835, he attended at the delivery of fourteen women, eight of whom developed puerperal fever and two of whom died. Answering Holmes's question, he admitted that he had not changed his outer coat until August 6, the date of confinement of the last victim. Holmes studied two other such remarkable clusters and reviewed all the published work in the field. In prose that achieves clarity and grandeur he reported his conclusions:

> I am too much in earnest for either humility or vanity, but I do entreat those who hold the keys of life and death to listen to me also for this once. I ask no personal favor; but I beg to be heard in behalf of the women whose lives are at stake, until some stronger voice shall plead for them. . . . The practical point to be illustrated is the following: *The disease known as Puerperal Fever is so far contagious as to be frequently carried from patient to patient by physicians and nurses.* [Holmes's italics]

When the precautions he urged were applied in practice, childbirth became safer in Massachusetts.

Holmes's discovery had two far-reaching consequences. With respect to medical science, it has been ranked with Morton's discovery of anesthesia (1846) and Beaumont's discovery of the digestive action of the stomach (1836) as one of the three great achievements of nineteenth-century American medicine. With respect to the sanitary revolution, it was a political act of self-criticism that permitted American medicine to become regarded as a learned profession devoted to the public good rather than as a guild protecting its perquisites. Oliver Wendell Holmes achieved in life that which Tertius Lydgate never quite managed in *Middlemarch*, a discovery which Eliot would certainly have described as "the union of intellectual conquest with social good." Holmes made that discovery by applying his imagination—and rhetoric—to the quantitative analysis of case records that he had learned from Louis. And medical literature from Holmes's *The Contagiousness of Puerperal Fever* to this week's issue of *The New England Journal of Medicine* unites detection and observation, riddle and solution, medicine and meliorism.

As for his literary endeavors, so much an aspect of his medical imagination and rhetoric, the verdict of his longtime editor, William Dean Howells, seems to have been the verdict of posterity: "He was not a man who cared to transcend; he liked bounds, he liked horizons, the constancy of shores. He did not discover new continents . . . but men as great and as useful as [Columbus] stayed behind and found an America of the mind without straying from their thresholds." That summary was written at the end of Holmes's life when he was merely a well-known literary figure. But when the young Holmes *had* strayed from his threshold to cross the Atlantic, he brought back seeds of a discovery that did, in fact, "transcend." Purely literary folk underestimate the cultural bounds, horizons, and constancy of

shores that permitted *The Contagiousness of Puerperal Fever*
and "The Chambered Nautilus" to issue from one pen.

Among the books Holmes brought home with him from
Paris were copies of Keats's poems and the collected works of
Thomas Browne. They were examples to him of how literature
and medicine could coexist as the passions of one man. Browne's
Religio Medici had caught his particular attention because of
Browne's notion of the hospital as a pesthouse. Before the rise
of secular philanthropy in the eighteenth century, hospitals were
houses of God to which the ill repaired for terminal care. No
one prepared a record, registered the signs and symptoms of
disease, or probed into the personal history of a patient. Nor,
one might add, had the novel or murder mystery been dreamed
of. Sir Thomas reminds us of the narrative genres available to
him: "Now for my life, it is a miracle of thirty years, which to
relate, were not a History, but piece of Poetry, and would sound
to common ears like a fable. For the World, I count it not an
Inn, but an Hospital; and a place not to live, but to die in."

Two centuries later, John Keats concluded that the world was
a teaching hospital after eight months of trudging the wards as
an apothecary student and after twelve months as a surgical
dresser at Guy's Hospital, to which more than ten thousand
patients were admitted every year: "I will call the world a School
instituted for the purpose of teaching. . . . Do you not see how
necessary a World of Pains and troubles is to school an Intelligence and make it a soul?"

In the World of Pains and troubles, Keats's world of Guy's
and St. Thomas's Hospitals, the narrative was a case record in
which the plot of diagnosis had been distilled from hundreds of
similar narratives. When Dr. Holmes read Browne confessing
that his world is a hospital, Holmes must have heard the stern
voice of a seventeenth-century conscience. But when Keats,
writing at the dawn of the Romantic era, assured his fellows that
the world is a school for the purpose of teaching, he heard the
fluttering of meliorist wings. The doctor's soul—that urge for

social good—must be weaned from mere intelligence by the experience of pains and troubles. That experience was written down in case records.

Since the Paris of 1830 and the Boston of 1834, those records have contained as much science as a text by Cuvier or the "open reading frame" of a modern gene. Even when kept by lesser scribes than Oliver Wendell Holmes, the purpose of those records is no less noble than that of imaginative literature. They are meant to school our intelligence and make it a soul. Medicine and literature share that moral function, which may be worth reconsidering now that most of us seem to believe that the world is more like an inn than a hospital.

3. DR. BLACKWELL RETURNS FROM LONDON

You ask, what use will she make of her liberty when she has so long been sustained and restrained? I answer in the first place this will not be suddenly given. . . . But were this freedom to come suddenly, I have no fear of the consequences. . . . If you ask me what offices they may fill, I reply—any. I do not care what case you put; let them be sea captains if they will. I do not doubt there are women fitted for such an office . . .

—Margaret Fuller, *Woman in the Nineteenth Century*, 1845

As we shall see in the next chapter, Margaret Fuller and her husband and infant son were drowned by shipwreck on July 19, 1850, when an inexperienced sea captain ran the ship they were traveling in aground on a sandbar off Fire Island. Exactly one year later, another American woman returned to America from postgraduate medical studies in London to a reception only somewhat more hospitable than Fuller's. Dr. Elizabeth Blackwell (1821–1910), described by *The Lancet* as "the first woman medical graduate in the modern meaning of the phrase," arrived in New York to set up medical practice. She, too, found her medical vocation at the École de Médecine where Dr. Holmes had studied, while her life in reform realized George Eliot's hope that the profession would combine the goals of intellectual conquest with social good. In several aspects Dr. Blackwell's career paralleled that of Dr. Holmes. Children of preachers, both had imbibed the sternest of Puritan values, both softened their views in the light of French culture, both lived in the service of public hygiene. Both strongly opposed the heresies of Mesmer and homeopathy, and both strongly believed that meliorist reason would "increase the power of positive good" in the new republic.

Born in England to Samuel Blackwell, a well-off sugar refiner and dissident lay preacher, she and her eight siblings were brought to live in Cincinnati, where family friends soon included both Henry Ward Beecher and Harriet Beecher Stowe. Her exposure to Unitarian thought in Cincinnati and to Quaker physicians in Philadelphia turned her interests to medicine, and she received medical tutorials in the private practices of friendly doctors. Despite thorough preparation in anatomy classes and a solid educational record, she was refused admission by every medical faculty in Philadelphia, New York City, and Boston, and by Bowdoin and Yale.

However, there was a small medical faculty in Geneva, New York, that was empowered to give the degree of Doctor of Medicine, provided lectures were attended for two years and a thesis was written. The Geneva school requirements for the M.D. degree were par for the course, as it were, and the faculty put the question of a woman's admission to the students of the little upstate school; to their credit, the young men passed the following two resolutions, a copy of which remained with Blackwell to her death:

1. *Resolved:* That one of the radical principles of a Republican Government is the universal education of both sexes; that to every branch of scientific education the doors should be open equally to all; that the application of Elizabeth Blackwell to become a member of our class meets our entire approbation; and in extending our unanimous invitation we pledge ourselves that no conduct of ours shall cause her to regret her attendance at this institution.

2. *Resolved:* That a copy of these proceedings be signed by
the chairman and transmitted to Elizabeth Blackwell.

In the event, she matriculated in November 1846, was more or
less well received by town and gown, and performed splendidly
in all her courses, especially therapeutics. In the summer of 1848,
she took her clinical instruction at the Philadelphia Hospital,
where an epidemic of typhus—or typhoid—was in progress.
This outbreak in an Irish immigrant population prompted her
to collect the records of its victims and to describe how it was
spread from case to case; the account became her doctoral thesis.
Recommending light, air, and soap, her small treatise is only
somewhat less professional than Holmes's on puerperal fever.
Blackwell's thesis also relied on the work Dr. Charles Louis,
quoting his 1829 book on the distinction between typhus and
typhoid. (That is the volume, we recall from *Middlemarch*, to
which Lydgate turns before he gives up his dreams of research
to marry Rosamond Vincy.) By February 1849, Blackwell's thesis had been published in the *Buffalo Medical Journal and Review*, and all that remained for her doctorate was to finish the
two-year course of study, which she did with distinction. Her
younger brother Henry—of whom more later—described the
scene of her graduation:

> The President taking off his hat rose, and addressing her in
> the same formula [as the others but] substituting *Domina for
> Domine*, presented her the diploma, whereupon our Sis, who
> had walked up and stood before him with much dignity,
> bowed and half turned to retire, but suddenly turning back
> replied: "Sir, I thank you; by the help of the Most High it
> shall be the effort of my life to shed honor upon your
> diploma."

The occasion was an event in both the United States and England, and the press by and large commented favorably. London's

Punch chimed in with lines that would have made Rosamond Vincy cringe:

> *Young ladies all, of every clime*
>   *Especially in Britain,*
> *Who wholly occupy your time*
>   *In novels or in knitting,*
> *Whose highest skill is but to play*
>   *Sing, dance, or French to clack well,*
> *Reflect on the example, pray,*
>   *Of excellent Miss Blackwell!*
>
> *For Doctrix Blackwell—that's the way*
>   *To dub in rightful gender—*
> *In her profession, ever may*
>   *Prosperity attend her!*
> *'Punch' a gold-handled parasol*
>   *Suggests for presentation*
> *To one so well deserving all*
>   *Esteem and admiration.*

The degree won, Blackwell determined to become a surgeon. She was advised to seek the best clinical training possible and told that France was the place to obtain it. As we have seen, young American doctors properly regarded Paris as the fount of clinical science, and plucky Blackwell sailed off to the City of Light. Her adventures in Paris and afterward are described in a sparkling memoir, *Pioneer Work in Opening the Medical Profession to Women*, a volume that can stand comfortably on the shelf of meliorist literature somewhere between Thomas Wentworth Higginson's *Army Life in a Black Regiment* and *Middlemarch*. Blackwell picked Paris as

the one place where I should be able to find unlimited opportunities for study in any branch of the medical art. . . . On May 21, 1849, with a very slender purse and few intro-

ductions of any value, I found myself in the unknown world
of Paris, bent upon the one object of pursuing my studies,
with no idea of the fierce political passions then smoldering
amongst the people, nor with any fear of the cholera which
was then threatening an epidemic.

Like young Oliver Wendell Holmes, who had come after the
July Revolution of 1830, she arrived in the middle of social unrest; like Holmes, she was thrilled by French sights and sounds;
unlike Holmes, her first purchase was a new bonnet, "choosing
plain grey silk, although I was assured again and again that nobody wore that color." Blackwell required a new bonnet because, again unlike Holmes, she was no unknown quantity; and
her few introductions of any value included one to the poet
Alphonse Lamartine, the short-term head of the short-term Second Republic. Tocqueville had said of him, "I do not think that
I ever met in the world of ambitious egoists in which I lived
any mind so untroubled by thought of the common good as
his." Blackwell was only somewhat more impressed:

> I was asked if I was a lady from America, for Lamartine is to
> most people *in the country*. I was shown through several ante-
> chambers into a drawing-room, where stood the poet enter-
> taining some visitors, he bowed, requested me to wait a few
> moments and withdrew to his apartment: a lofty room, carved
> and richly gilded, three long windows opening on to a bal-
> cony and commanding a garden full of trees. The room con-
> tained a rich carpet and purple velvet couches, some portraits,
> an exquisite female profile in bas-relief, a golden chandelier
> from the ceiling, some antique vases, etc. and a soft green light
> from the trees of the large garden suffused the room.

Lamartine received her with Gallic poise, appearing "very tall
and slender, but the most graceful man I have ever seen, every

movement was like music; grey eyes and hair." Blackwell transmitted messages to him from friends in Philadelphia of the
French Republic; Lamartine made amiable chatter in English—
his wife was English—and said he was pleased to have these
expressions of solidarity from friends of reform overseas. "There
was perfect harmony in the man and his surroundings. Doubt-
less he is a true man, though unable to work into practice the
great thoughts he cherishes." So went the meeting between the
liberal poet-politician of France and the first Anglo-Saxon female physician. (Her book makes livelier reading these days than
his poems.)

The next letter brought to her door none other than Dr. Louis
himself, "then at the height of his reputation." She felt instinctively that his visit was one of inspection. She told him she was
in need of practical work in surgery, and after a long conversation he informed her of what she must do to be permitted to
work at the Maternité, where she would in a very short time
become expert in "one small field of surgery, obstetrics and gy-
necology." Shortly thereafter and with Louis's intervention, she
was admitted in the autumn of 1849 for a six-month course.

In the enclosed world of the Maternité teaching and practice
were conducted by midwives (*sages-femmes*) in a conventlike
atmosphere supervised by men. Her most intellectually stimu-
lating companion was neither a midwife nor the professor in
charge but the intern M. Hippolyte Blot. They exchanged lessons in English and histology, spending hours at the young
man's microscope:

> By such examination different formations can be distin-
> guished from each other; thus cancer possesses very distinc-
> tive elements. It is necessary to examine bodies of varying
> shapes under different foci of the microscope, otherwise il-
> lusions may be created. In illustration he placed some blood
> globules and showed us that what appeared to be a central

spot in each globule was owing to the convexity not being in focus, and it disappeared when the focus was a little lengthened.

He is busy himself now in preparing for an examination of *internes*; if he gains the gold medal, he has the right to enter any hospital he chooses as an *interne* for a second term, and receive also his M.D., not otherwise granted to an *interne*. What chance have women shut out from these instructions? Work on, Elizabeth!

Today M. Blot spoke of a friend, Claude Bernard, a distinguished young inquirer, who is now, he thinks, on the eve of a discovery that will immortalize him . . . of the power which the liver has of secreting sugar in a normal state when animals are fed on certain substances which can be so converted; also of the curious experiment by which a dog was made, in his presence, to secrete albuminous or diabetic urine.

Claude Bernard (1813–78), who may be called the founder of experimental medicine, once remarked that science is like a brilliantly lighted banquet hall which can only be reached after walking through a warren of ghastly and ill-lit kitchens. Young Drs. Blot and Blackwell were in no bright hall at the Maternité. They were like Rosencrantz and Guildenstern in a Denmark of physiological chemistry, and Bernard's finding that blood sugar came from liver glycogen (glycogenolysis) was a towering Elsinore of mid-century science. The discovery of glycogenolysis, which led to an understanding of sugar and energy metabolism as well as of diabetes, did in fact make the "young inquirer" immortal, and one can construct a line of descent from Claude Bernard to the heroes of modern molecular biology—to James Watson and Francis Crick, François Jacob and Jacques Monod, David Baltimore and Paul Berg and Jim Bishop and Harold Varmus.

With her appetite for the new, young Dr. Blackwell in Paris tasted not only real science but also the mock. On a rare day off from the *sages-femmes*, she visited her sister Anna, who was living with another young American woman on the rue Fleurus (a street destined to become popular with American women: it was the future home of Gertrude Stein and Alice B. Toklas). From there the sisters went to a magnetic séance at the atelier of a socialite mesmerist, the Baron Dupotet. He, too, was at the height of his power, having recently converted half the alienists of England to the cause of what was to be called "hypnosis."

The Blackwells were brought to a large, darkened room at the top floor of a large house on the Ile de la Cité. A great portrait of Mesmer himself dominated the antechamber of the Baron's quarters, its frame encrusted with firebrands and anchors and other significant images; he looked fixedly at a pale lady opposite to him who had evidently undergone several magnetic crises. A great number of indecipherable verses were tacked to the walls or hanging from the ceiling. In this large waiting room, a shifting population of fifty or so people went to and fro. This included a lady with a hole in her cheek, the painter to the King of Sweden, the son of the English consul in Sicily, and "a remarkable fat dame, seated just within the folding-doors, who had powerful fits of nervous twitching, which gave her a singular appearance of pale tremulous red jelly." The Baron's inner chamber was smaller and ornamented by mystic symbols and black letter books of the Black Art. There was housed the inevitable oval metallic mirror "traced with magic characters which exerts a truly wonderful effect upon impressionable subjects, exciting an ecstasy of delight or a transport of rage." One or another of the crowd would rush to grab it from the mesmerist; small amiable spats broke out over its possession.

No miracles were wrought that day, Blackwell assures us. Nevertheless the faithful audience hung with great interest on every example of hypnotism: "the aspiring features assumed a higher aspect, the downward ones bent more determinedly, and the red jelly became more tremulous at every fresh magnetization; and when the *séance* closed everybody shook everybody's hand, and found it good to have been there." Blackwell judged the Baron an honest man who for twenty-five years had been pursuing difficult and arcane subjects; "how much truth he may possess I am quite unable to say, for my position . . . has given me no power of really investigating them."

Back with her patients at the Maternité for only a few days, a very grave accident befell Dr. Blackwell: "in the dark early morning, whilst syringing the eye of one of my tiny patients for purulent ophthalmia," some of the water spurted into her left eye. By nightfall on November 4, the eye had become swollen, and by the next morning, the lids were "closely adherent from suppuration." The diagnosis of purulent ophthalmia, the dreaded venereal disease of newborns and those who attended them, was made by a young staff physician, and the twenty-eight-year-old Blackwell was placed in the student infirmary.

We now know that the disease is caused by the gonococcus, is due to chronic gonorrheal infection of the female reproductive tract, and was part of the load borne by the prostitutes and working women who gave birth in the public hospitals of Paris. The bacteriological revolution has all but eliminated it, but Albert Neisser did not discover the microbe until 1879, and it was not until 1884 that Karl Credé showed that eyedrops of 1% silver nitrate on the lids of newborns were an effective prophylactic. Thanks to rigorous maternal health laws, by the turn of the century prophylaxis had pretty much eliminated neonatal ophthalmia from advanced countries; today, unfortunately, it is making a comeback in Africa and Asia. But this was 1849, and Elizabeth Blackwell was treated by accepted methods of the day: cauterization of the lids, leeches to the temple, cold compresses, ointment of belladonna, opium to the forehead, purgatives, and footbaths. She was placed on a broth diet, and the eye was syringed every hour. "I realized the danger of the disease from the weapons employed against it," she remembered. Her friend M. Blot consulted his chief and he was given permission to devote the first days of the illness entirely to her case. He came in every two hours, day and night, to tend the eye. But despite his efforts, after three days it became obvious to her doctors that the eye was hopelessly infected. "Ah! how dreadful it was to find the daylight gradually fading as my kind doctor bent over me and removed with an exquisite delicacy of touch the films that had formed over the pupil! I could see him for a moment clearly, but the sight soon vanished, and the eye was left in darkness."

She lay in bed with both eyes closed for three weeks, but then the right eye gradually began to open and she could start to do little things for herself. She immediately wrote to her uncle, an English army officer—her father had died in Cincinnati when she was much younger—assuring him of her resolution to continue her career in medicine. "I beg uncle to feel quite sure that a brave soldier's niece will never disgrace the colours she fights under but will be proud of the wounds gained in a great cause." She downplayed her injury and told him that the accident could have been worse—the left eye was not greatly disfigured and would in time appear less so. She finished her letter with the assurance that she could write without difficulty, read a little, and hoped very soon to return to her studies. "I certainly esteem myself very fortunate and still mean to be at no very distant day *the first lady surgeon in the world.*"

As soon as she was up and about, she conspired with her sister to find a present for M. Blot, whose constant attention and compassion touched her deeply. "My friendship deepened for my young physician, and I planned a little present for his office." A very elegant pair of lamps were secured by Anna, which Blackwell, "bundled up in my dressing gown and shawl, looking and feeling very much like a ghost," hurried through the corridors to receive. That night she brought the lamps to Blot's consultation room, and in the morning, the young intern "came to me evidently full of delight, and longing to be amiable, yet too conscientious to infringe the rules of the Maternité by acknowledging the present." She was discharged on November

26 permanently blind in one eye. Despite her passionate ambition to be "the first lady surgeon in the world," because of this handicap she disqualified herself from surgery or obstetrics as a career.

She went to various spas in Germany to convalesce, and while there resolved to continue her training in medicine. She applied to St. Bartholomew's Hospital in London, then perhaps the strongest teaching hospital of the city. The illustrious English physician Sir James Paget endorsed her admission as a student "in the wards and other departments of the hospital," and on May 14 she was accepted at Bart's. Once on the wards, her zeal for medical science was as high and her dreams of reform as ambitious as those of any Lydgate or Holmes. She soon spotted the difference between the medicine of Paris and London at mid-century:

> I do not find so active a spirit of investigation in the English professors as in the French. In Paris this spirit pervaded young and old, and gave a wonderful fascination to the study of medicine, which even I, standing on the threshold, strongly felt. There are innumerable medical societies there, and some of the members are always *on the eve* of most important discoveries; a brilliant theory is *almost* proved, and creates intense interest; some new plan of treatment is always exciting attention in the hospitals, and its discussion is widely spread by the immense crowds of students freely admitted.

But Bart's had its pleasures as well. Blackwell was courteously treated, saw the best of empiric medicine, and walked with men who, while not experimental or quantitative in approach, still felt clinical medicine in their sinews and knew how to examine patients. She wrote to her sister:

> This famous old hospital is only five minutes' walk from my lodgings, and every morning as the clock strikes nine, I walk

down Holborn Hill, make a short cut through the once famous Cock Lane, and find myself at a gate of the hospital
that enables me to enter with only a side glance at Smithfield
Cattle Market . . . Mr. Paget spoke to the students before I
joined the class. When I entered and bowed, I received a
round of applause. My seat is always reserved for me and I
have no trouble. There are so many physicians and surgeons,
so many wards, and all so exceedingly busy, that I have not
yet got the run of the place; but the medical wards are thrown
open unreservedly to me either to follow the physician's visits
or for private study.

She also saw some of the same mock science that had flourished in France: mesmerism, homeopathy, and hydropathy,
which she called the three heresies to distinguish them from the
old system. But, after looking into the heresies a little more
closely, she felt as dissatisfied with them as with what she had
been taught: "We hear of such wonderful cures constantly being
wrought by this and the other thing, that we forget on how
small a number the novelty has been exercised, and the failures
are never mentioned; but on the same principle, I am convinced
that if the old system were the heresy, and the heresy the established custom, we should hear the same wonders related of the
drugs." There is more than an echo here of Holmes's "If all the
Materia Medica as now used, could be sunk to the bottom,—it
would be the better for mankind and all the worse for the
fishes." Sound advice in the days before penicillin.

Her mentor gave her some advice, which elicited a passionate
response:

Mr. Paget who is very cordial, tells me that I shall have to
encounter much more prejudice from ladies than from gentlemen in my course. I am prepared for this. Prejudice is more
violent the blinder it is, and I think Englishwomen seem wonderfully shut up in their habitual views. But a work of the

ages cannot be hindered by individual feeling. A hundred years hence women will not be what they are now.

Blackwell's experiences in Paris and London made her eager to start out on her own in America. She wrote of her future plans to her sister Emily in November 1850. Emily had decided to follow in her sister's footsteps and was being privately tutored by Dr. John Davis, an anatomy demonstrator in Cincinnati:

> Here I have been following now with earnest attention, for a few weeks, the practice of a very large London hospital, and I find that the majority of patients do get well; so I have come to this conclusion—that I must begin with a practice which is an old established custom, which has really more expressed science than any other system (the three heresies) but nevertheless, as it dissatisfies me heartily, I shall commence as soon as possible building a hospital in which I can experiment; and the very instant I feel *sure* of any improvement I shall adopt it in my practice, in spite of a whole legion of opponents . . . I advise you E. to familiarize yourself with the healthy sound of the chest. I wish I could lend you my little black stethoscope that I brought from the Maternité.

When she returned to New York she was too poor to realize the dream of building an experimental hospital. "If I were rich," she had told her sister, "I would not begin private practice, but would only experiment. As however I am poor, I have no choice." Choice absent, she went about doing God's work on earth. She set up a general practice and spent cold winters and steaming summers trudging the pavements with her black bag. Work on, Elizabeth! Proudly sporting the stethoscope she had brought from the Maternité, she attended to mainly poor, mainly female, chiefly immigrant patients. Her early years as this nation's first woman doctor of medicine were not encouraging. She confessed her deep unhappiness: "I had no medical com-

panionship, the profession stood aloof, and society was distrust-
ful of the innovation. Insolent letters occasionally came by post,
and my pecuniary position was a source of constant anxiety."
It was impossible to rent an office, the term "female physician"
having been preempted by ill-trained abortionists, and she went
into debt by buying a house on East Fifteenth Street. She
worked in the attic and the basement, renting out the remainder
of the house. Her isolation prompted her to adopt a seven-year-
old orphan, Katharine Barry, and this young child grew into a
lifetime companion, friend, and housekeeper.

Slowly, Elizabeth Blackwell began to attract support from the
New York Quaker community, and in 1854 she opened on the
Lower East Side a one-room dispensary in which she treated
more than two hundred women in the first year. Its first annual
report, written to rouse further support, spelled out its aims:

> The design of this institution is to give to poor women the op-
> portunity of consulting physicians of their own sex. The ex-
> isting charities of our city regard the employment of women
> as physicians as an experiment, the success of which has not
> been sufficiently proved to admit of cordial co-operation. It
> was therefore necessary to provide for a separate institution
> which should furnish to poor women the medical aid which
> they could not obtain elsewhere.

By 1856, the sisters were reunited. Emily had also had extensive medical training after having earned an M.D. degree from
Western Reserve. She had walked the wards of Bellevue in New
York, and spent two *Wanderjahre* working with Sir James Young
Simpson in Edinburgh, Franz von Winckel in Dresden, and William Jenner at the Children's Hospital in London. The Blackwell
pluck and persistence paid off. Elizabeth's goal of founding an
experimental hospital was achieved, but the medical experiments
performed in it were in the field of women's rights and social
justice rather than physiology or therapeutics. With the help of

progressive philanthropists and their good friend Horace Greeley, the Blackwells established in 1857 the New York Infirmary
for Women and Children at 64 Bleecker Street. They success-
fully overcame every objection of the time: that female doctors
would require police protection on their rounds; that only male
resident physicians could control the patients, that "classes and
persons" might be admitted whom "it would be an insult to
treat" (i.e., beggars and prostitutes); that signatures on death
certificates might be invalid (the legal rights of women in the
presuffrage era were fragile); that the male trustees might be held
responsible for any "accidents"; and that in any case no one
would supply women with enough money to support such an
unpopular effort.

With Emily in charge of this going concern, Elizabeth traveled back to England and became the first woman to be registered as a physician in that country. She studied programs of
maternal hygiene, looked over public-health programs for
women and children, and toyed with the notion of spending the
rest of her life founding a country hospital with Florence Nightingale, to whom she had formed an intense personal attachment.
The delicate overtones of her memoir anticipate lines that Katharine Lee Bates dedicated to Nightingale a generation later:

> *Fragrant thy name as the City of Flowers;*
> *Sweet thy name as a song in the night;*
> *Over all wonders of womanhood towers*
> *Thy glory, white as the Cross is white.*

When Elizabeth returned to New York in 1860, the sisters
enlarged the infirmary once more, added new staff, and put in
place the preventive measures of the sanitarian revolution. Their
most critical innovations were in community health; they were
the first to send "sanitary visitors" to the poorer neighborhoods
of the city; their Tenement House Service was the earliest in-
stance of medical social service in the United States.

The Civil War engaged the abolitionist spirit of the Blackwell family. On the day after Fort Sumter was fired on, the Black-wells helped to found the National Sanitary Aid Society; this later became the nucleus of the Sanitary Commission. The Blackwells also acted as a conduit for the nursing corps which Dorothea Dix was assembling in Washington:

> All that could be done in the extreme urgency of the need was to sift out the most promising women from the multi-tudes that applied to be sent on as nurses, put them for a month for training at the great Bellevue Hospital of New York, which consented to receive relays of volunteers, pro-vide them with a small outfit and send them on for distri-bution to Miss Dix.

When the war was over and finances permitted, another dream of Elizabeth Blackwell was realized. In those long nights at the Maternité she had written, "What chance have women shut out from these instructions? Work on, Elizabeth!" It was nineteen years later before women could receive such instruc-tions in New York: in 1868 the Blackwells founded a modern medical college for women which by 1908, when it was ab-sorbed by the newly coeducational Cornell University Medical College, had graduated 394 women doctors. Work on, Eliza-beth, indeed! The faculty included such eminent female physi-cians as Mary Putnam Jacobi and Elizabeth Cushier, professor of gynecologic surgery. The laboratories for instruction in both basic and applied sciences were among the most up-to-date in the country, and the three-year curriculum exceeded in rigor much of what passed for medical education elsewhere. Elizabeth Blackwell became the first professor of hygiene, and it was due to her efforts and those of Emily, who succeeded her, that many of the leaders of the sanitarian revolution got their start at the Women's Medical College of the New York Infirmary for Women and Children.

Perhaps the most remarkable aspect of the Blackwell family record is not their sanitarian or abolitionist zeal, but the large swath the family cut in feminist history. If the James family seemed to have "a serpent in its blood"—in the phrase of William James—the Blackwells had a colt. But their sanguine temperament ran in a direction opposite to that of the saturnine Jameses. Nowadays when one speaks of "the Blackwells" one includes not only Elizabeth and Emily but a small tribe of reformers that spanned three generations. Of the twelve children of Samuel and Hannah Lane Blackwell, three died in infancy; Anna became a newspaper correspondent for Horace Greeley; Ellen developed into an author and artist; Emily and Elizabeth were doctors; and two of the brothers, Samuel and Henry, had even more public careers.

Samuel Blackwell married Antoinette Louisa Brown, who in 1853 was ordained as the first woman minister of a recognized denomination in the United States (Congregational). One of the few pulpits that offered her a guest appearance was that of the Universalist congregation in Worcester, Massachusetts, led by Thomas Wentworth Higginson—the Higginson who nurtured Emily Dickinson's verse and who became colonel of a black regiment of freed slaves in South Carolina. As Louisa Brown, the future Blackwell had worked in New York's prisons and hospitals and written accounts of their need for institutional reform published in Greeley's *Tribune* and later collected as *Shadows of Our Social System* (1856). Samuel Blackwell had sought her out at her upstate church precisely because of her writings. An abolitionist to the core, she became after the Civil War an ardent supporter of the suffrage movement, and both Blackwells were active in Julia Ward Howe's Association for the Advancement of Women.

Henry Browne Blackwell, himself an ardent abolitionist and Free-Soiler, married Lucy Stone, an Oberlin classmate of Louisa Brown Blackwell. A pioneer feminist, she insisted on keeping her own last name after marriage; women who adhered to this custom were for a while called "Lucy Stoners." At their wedding ceremony, on May 1, 1855, the Blackwells agreed on having read publicly a protest against the marriage laws then on the books. The protest was given wide circulation in an account by the minister who presided over the wedding: Thomas Wentworth Higginson. Henry, seven years her junior, had courted Lucy for two stormy years before finally winning her over by the courageous act of saving a fugitive black woman from her owners. After the Civil War, Lucy Stone, Henry Blackwell, and their daughter Alice edited the influential feminist periodical *The Women's Journal.* It became the official voice of the American Woman Suffrage Association which Lucy Stone and Julia Ward Howe formed in 1869. The final public speech that Lucy Stone delivered was at the Columbian Exposition in 1893, naturally enough at the Woman's Building so beloved by Katharine Lee Bates. It was Stone's last chance at alabaster; she dodged the tomb and continued the Blackwell record of firsts by becoming the first person to be cremated in New England.

The personal affairs of Elizabeth and Emily Blackwell remained as monogamous as those of their brothers. Aside from that passionate episode with Florence Nightingale, Elizabeth spent all of her life—the last thirty years in seaside retirement —with her adopted daughter and friend Kitty Barry. Emily and *her* lifelong companion, Dr. Elizabeth Cushier, spent twenty-eight happy years together in a Gramercy Park brownstone and on the coast of Maine.

It is difficult to find a group of men and women more enmeshed than the Blackwells in the great movements of the last century, to find a family more involved with intellectual conquest and social good. But many would argue that the Holmes family made as great a contribution to reform as the Blackwells. The two Oliver Wendell Holmeses, the Autocrat of the Breakfast Table and his son, an Associate Justice of the Supreme Court, took the Brahmin road in support of many of the Blackwell causes, and the written record they left behind is more glittering by far than that of the Blackwells. Holmes Jr. thrice shed blood for the Union, and the doctor caused many to shed tears for the cause. One Civil War passage from the elder Holmes sums up the political philosophy which he and the Blackwells espoused, and which his son was to make part of the common law:

> This Republic is the chosen home of *minorities*, of the lesser power in the presence of the greater. It is a common error to speak of our distinction as consisting in the rule of the majority. Majorities, the greater material powers, have always ruled before. The history of most countries has been that of majorities, mounted majorities, clad in iron, armed with death, treading down the tenfold more numerous minorities. In the old civilizations they root themselves like oaks in the soil; men must live in their shadow or cut them down. With us the majority is only the flower of the passing noon, and the minority is the bud which may open in the next morning's sun. We must be tolerant, for the thought which stammers on a single tongue today may organize itself in the growing consciousness of time, and come back to us like the voice of the multitudinous waves of the ocean on the morrow.

It is now a century and a half later, and while the condition of women is not what it was one hundred years ago, we can see that the thoughts that stammered on the Blackwell tongue were slow in organizing themselves. It was not until 1915 that the medical school of New York University consented to give its first faculty position to a woman, Dr. S. Josephine Baker, one of this century's pioneers of social medicine. Dr. Baker had graduated from the Women's Medical College of the New York Infirmary for Women and Children in 1895, and after a distinguished period of practical work, she became a lecturer in child hygiene at Bellevue Hospital:

They never allowed me to forget that I was the first woman ever to impose herself on the college. I stood down in a well with tiers of seats rising all around me, surgical-theater fashion, and the seats were filled with unruly, impatient, hard-boiled young men. I opened my mouth to begin the lecture. Instantly, before a syllable could be heard, they began to clap thunderously, deafeningly, grinning and pounding their palms together. Then the only possible way of saving my face occurred to me. I threw back my head and roared with laughter, laughing at them and with them at the same time—and they stopped, as if somebody had turned a switch. I began to lecture like mad before they changed their minds, and they heard me in dead silence to the end. But the moment I stopped at the end of the hour, that horrible clapping began again. Frightened and tired as I was from talking a solid hour against a gloweringly hostile audience, I fled at top speed. Every lecture I gave at Bellevue, from 1915 through to 1930, was clapped in and clapped out that way; not the spontaneous burst of real applause that can sound so heart-warming, but instead, the flat, contemptuous whacking rhythms with which the crowd at a baseball game walk an unpopular player in from the outfield.

We've come a long way since 1930, and these days the impediments to full equality in the profession are more likely to arise de facto than de jure, but unfortunately the verdicts of prejudice can be as stern as those of law. The medical and social causes to which the Blackwells, the Holmeses, the Stones, and the Bakers devoted themselves have by and large prevailed: abolition of slavery achieved, the Union preserved, sanitation promoted, infections curbed, child and maternal health protected by the state, women's rights in the profession moving slowly ahead. We *are* farther along than Elizabeth Blackwell hoped on her return from London. Women are not what they were one hundred years ago. Yet we are still some distance from realizing

her fondest hope, that of a social movement which would unite
the sexes under the banner of moral reform.

On December 1, 1850, Elizabeth Blackwell regretted she
could not attend the Convention for Women's Rights in
Worcester:

> But I feel a little perplexed by the main object of the Con-
> vention—Women's Rights. The great object of education has
> nothing to do with woman's rights or man's rights, but with
> the development of the human soul and body . . . My great
> dream is of a grand moral reform society, a wide movement
> of women in this matter; the remedy to be sought in every
> sphere of life . . . Education to change both the male and
> female perverted character; industrial occupation, including
> formation of a priesthood of women; colonial operations,
> clubs, homes, social unions, a true Press; and the whole com-
> bined that it could be brought to bear on any outrage or
> prominent evil.

George Eliot could have called that grand moral reform movement "meliorism"—and she did.

4. MARGARET FULLER RETURNS
FROM ROME

Thus far, no woman in the world has ever once spoken out her whole heart and her whole mind. The mistrust and disapproval of the vast bulk of society throttles us, as with two gigantic hands at our throats! We mumble a few weak words, and leave a thousand better ones unsaid. You let us write a little, it is true, on a limited range of subjects. But the pen is not for woman. Her power is too natural and immediate. It is with the living voice, alone, that she can compel the world to recognize the light of her intellect and the depth of her heart.

—Nathaniel Hawthorne, *The Blithedale Romance*, 1852

The words in the epigraph are spoken by Zenobia, a character in Hawthorne's roman à clef, but the sentiments are those of Margaret Fuller, on whom Zenobia was based. Fuller (1810–50) had won fame as a member of the Boston Transcendentalist Club, as editor with Emerson of *The Dial*, and as a literary and cultural critic on Horace Greeley's *New York Tribune*. She had also gained notice as author of America's first feminist manifesto, *Woman in the Nineteenth Century*. Like Zenobia, Margaret Fuller was a sometime dweller in the Brook Farm community of Transcendentalists. Like Zenobia, Fuller was indeed able to "compel the world to recognize the light of her intellect and the depth of her heart." Again like Zenobia, Fuller was destined to be valued more for her living voice than for the works of her pen. And finally, like Zenobia, Fuller died by drowning in the prime of life because a Yankee let her down. She was also undone by a weighty work of sculpture: Hiram Powers's larger-than-life-size marble figure of Calhoun.

Daniel Webster of Massachusetts and John C. Calhoun of South Carolina, the two great debating senators in the antebellum Congress, had died a decade before the war that both had feared. But whereas Webster's statue still stands in New York's Central Park, Calhoun's had a more bizarre fate. After the attack on Fort Sumter, Calhoun's statue was moved inland from its home in the harbor town of Charleston, South Carolina, to the state house in Columbia to prevent its destruction by naval gunfire. This was to no avail, since both building and statue were destroyed, as was much of the capital itself, by fire and explosions on the day following Sherman's occupation of the town in 1865. To this day it remains unclear who set the blaze; Sherman and a postwar board of inquiry blamed the Confederate commander, Wade Hampton, for beginning the fire by torching bales of cotton to deny them to the Union. But "unintentional" fires seemed to accompany Sherman's entire campaign and even Ulysses Grant seemed less than certain of Sherman's role. As he wrote in his memoirs, "There has since been a great deal of acrimony displayed in discussions of the question as to who set Columbia on fire. . . . In any case, the example set by the Confederates in burning the village of Chambersburg, Pennsylvania, a town which was not garrisoned, would seem to make a defense of the act of firing the seat of government of the State most responsible for the conflict then raging, not imperative." The destruction of Columbia destroyed Powers's *Calhoun*. But earlier, *Calhoun* played a major role in Margaret Fuller's death.

Only after her death were the men and women of the Boston Enlightenment aware that they had lost America's first international woman of letters. Julia Ward Howe said of her in retrospect, "Her figure would appropriately guard the entrance of the enlarged domain of womanhood of which she was the inspired pythoness." But Fuller had her own sense of the temple, and her journal in 1839 records this pre-Freudian fantasy: "This destiny of the thinker, and (shall I dare say it) of the poetic priestess, sibylline, dwelling in the cave, or amid the Libyan sands, lay yet enfolded in my mind. Accordingly, I did not look on any of the persons, brought into relation with me, with common womanly eyes."

This exalted sense of self, the "sense that the priestess must reserve her paeans for Apollo," did not endear her to all of America's literary lions. Nor did her avowal to Carlyle that "she had seen all the people worth seeing in America and was satisfied that there was no intellect comparable to her own" sit well with other claimants to the title. James Russell Lowell, insulted by her criticism, complained of her egotism and her

> . . . I turn-the-crank-of-the-Universe air
> And a tone, which at least to my fancy, appears
> Not so much to be entering as boxing your ears,
> Is unfolding a tale (of herself, I surmise,
> For 't is dotted as thick as a peacock with I's).

Emerson termed her obsession with self an attempt to climb the "mountain *me*," and in England, Carlyle recognized her "predetermination to *eat* this big universe as her oyster or her egg." In hindsight, many of us who have had a chance to read her collected works recently are more inclined to accept Fuller's self-evaluation than the put-downs of her friends and rivals.

Fuller lived in Europe for four years before she laid eyes on Powers's *Calhoun*. She served as a foreign correspondent for the *Tribune*—another female first—becoming more and more involved in the politics of the European left. She met with George Sand, William Wordsworth, Harriet Martineau, and Dr. Southwood Smith—a physician who pioneered public housing and who kept the skeleton of Jeremy Bentham in his study. She also became great friends with Giuseppe Mazzini, leader of the Roman Republic. In her Roman years, she lived high adventure, slipped to deep depression, and finally married a younger Italian, a handsome but ignorant stud named Giovanni Angelo, Marquis Ossoli, by whom she bore a late-in-life child.

The marriage was unusual at best. Fuller did not inform her mother until a year after the fact:

> The first moment, it may cause you a pang to know that your eldest child might long ago have been addressed by another name than yours, and has a little son a year old . . . My husband is a Roman and of a noble but impoverished house. He is not in any respect such a person as people in general would expect to find with me; and of that which is contained in books, he is absolutely ignorant, and he has no enthusiasm of character.

Notwithstanding these differences, Ossoli and Fuller lived happily enough until time and reduced circumstances forced them to go back to her native land.

Hawthorne used Ossoli as a model for his Italian hero in *The Marble Faun*, unwisely naming him Donatello. He provides a sympathetic view of the disparate marriage between Fuller and Ossoli:

> People of high intellectual endowments do not require similar ones in those they love. They are just the persons to appreciate the wholesome gush of feeling, the honest affection, the simple joy, the fullness of contentment with what he loves, which Miriam sees in Donatello. True; she may call him a simpleton. It is a necessity of the case, for a man loses the capacity for this kind of affection, in proportion as he cultivates and refines himself.

Ossoli fought bravely on the barricades for the Roman Republic against the royalist-papal armies of France and Austria during the Revolution of 1848–49. Fuller, now the Marquesa

Ossoli, and afire with the "blood-colours of Socialistic views," as Elizabeth Barrett Browning described them, lent all her energy to the republican cause, and dispatched glowing accounts of the Republic's virtues to the *Tribune*. She also sent her baby out of danger to a wet nurse in Rieti and freed herself to work day and night as a volunteer nurse in the Tiber Island hospitals. In those bloody field stations, as the American chargé later described, "the weather was intensely hot; her health was feeble and delicate; the dead and dying were around her in every stage of pain and horror."

After fleeing to exile in Florence, the couple found little peace, though they found several friendly doors open in the Anglo-American colony of upper bohemians, many of whom had also fled from Rome. Fuller's friends and benefactors included not only Robert and Elizabeth Barrett Browning, but also the American sculptors William Wetmore Story, Thomas Crawford, and Horace Greenough (brother-in-law of Julia Ward Howe). And then there was Hiram Powers, at the peak of his reputation, putting the finishing touches on his *Calhoun*.

The subject of the *Calhoun* statue gives us a virtual text on the issues of antebellum American democracy. Twice Vice President and once Secretary of War, Calhoun stood at one end of an honorable North-South dialectic in the era before the Civil War; Webster held fast at the other. But whereas the Yankee pleaded for "Liberty and Union, Now and Forever, One and Inseparable!" Calhoun's counter-slogan was designed to remind slave owners of the legal basis for states' rights. Powers's statue showed Calhoun clad in a Roman toga, bare left arm uplifted, holding a great scroll upon which his motto was carved in stone: "Truth, Justice, and the Constitution." His right arm rested on a fasces-like palmetto, the state tree of South Carolina. At the harbor of Charleston, in the garb of a Roman senator, a marble Calhoun would make his last stand, his statue the guardian of agrarian rights. There was some hurry. Calhoun, the great champion of the Southern way, had died in March and the statue was to be his Charleston monument: a piece of public art in service to the state.

A distraught Margaret Fuller was afraid that the Austrians, who controlled Tuscany, would detain her politically suspect husband or perhaps harm their child, now a year and a half old; accounts of Austro-Croat atrocities in Lombardy were current. She borrowed money from friends for the cheapest passage home: it was on the bark *Elizabeth*, out of Livorno. On May 2, 1850, she wrote from Florence to the American chargé in Rome: "I sail in the barque *Elizabeth* for New York. She is laden with marble and rags—a very appropriate companionship for wares of Italy! She carries Powers' statue of Calhoun. Adieu!"

Filled with anxiety over the ocean voyage—no mean crossing in a three-master—she also wrote to a friend: "I am absurdly fearful, and various omens have combined to give me a dark feeling. I am become indeed a miserable coward for the sake of [my child]. I fear heat and cold, even moschetoes [sic], fear terribly the voyage home, fear biting poverty . . ."

Over most of her life, Fuller had depended on the kindness of strangers. In the days when she supported her fatherless family by work as a schoolmistress in Boston, she had written: "I have no home on earth . . . but driven from home to home, I get the picture and poetry of each. Keys of gold, silver, iron and lead are in my casket. No one loves me."

So, off to America on the *Elizabeth* sailed the socialist, penniless Marquis and Marquesa Ossoli with tons of marble and John C. Calhoun in the hold. The first six days out of Livorno went well; the weather was fair and little Angelo was the pet of all on board. But soon after Fuller's fortieth birthday— May 23—things turned sour. Captain Hardy, a Yankee salt, took sick of smallpox and died rapidly as the ship hove to off Gibraltar on June 2. The bark spent a week in quarantine and Fuller was able to dispatch a letter—her last—in which she worried that her dear child might catch the disease. She and Ossoli were immune, she believed, but:

In the earlier days, before I suspected smallpox, I carried him [Angelo] twice into the sick room, at the request of the captain . . . who was becoming fond of him. It is vain, by prudence, to seek to evade the stern assaults of destiny. I submit. Should all end well, we shall be in New York later than I expected; but keep a look-out . . . adieu, and love as you can, your friend,

Margaret

The stern assaults of destiny struck shortly after the bark took sail on June 9; the child came down with a mild case of the disease. Happily, he recovered, and the Ossolis became for a short while carefree on the voyage. The Marquis took vigorous if unsuccessful language instruction from a fellow passenger, Margaret wrote, and her son made a playfellow of a shipboard goat. The first mate, a Mr. Bangs, was now skipper; the winds were good and by noon of July 18 the boat was off the New Jersey shore. That evening Mr. Bangs had the passengers prepare for disembarkment in the morning.

In the middle of the night a gale blew up. Waves and wind drove the ship shoreward. In an effort to avoid Sandy Hook, a spit of land before New York Harbor, Bangs put the *Elizabeth* on an east-northeast course under close-reefed sails (the details are from contemporary accounts). But the inexperienced commander was driven farther along toward Long Island, and at four in the morning the *Elizabeth* ran aground on a sandbar. They were within a few hundred yards of Fire Island. It was then that the heavy marble—Calhoun, his pedestal, and chunks of Carrara stone—acted as a kind of internal battering ram as the waves banged them into timber and shattered the hold. Without that marble aboard, observers reckoned, the hull would have remained intact. It took twelve hours for the ship to fall apart completely. By daybreak, the trapped passengers could see a lifeboat on the shore, but the gale and surf did not permit its launch. Eventually, even the forecastle, to which the survivors had retreated, fell apart. Some of the crewmen swam ashore, Fuller was able to hand little Angelo into the arms of a steward—and then a huge wave dashed everyone away. Twenty minutes later, the bodies of the steward and little Angelo washed ashore; the bodies of Fuller and her husband were never recovered. Days later, her old friend Henry David Thoreau wandered the sands looking for remnants of the Ossolis, but nothing else had washed ashore.

Margaret Fuller and her husband survive as citizens in the republic of letters: she became Zenobia in *The Blithedale Romance*, Miriam in *The Marble Faun*, and Elsie Venner in Holmes's first novel, named after her character. Ossoli was—dare one say?—recast as *The Marble Faun*. The marble *Calhoun* was reborn more promptly: a public subscription made it possible to salvage the statue, which was recovered intact except for that broken left arm with its faithful motto. Soon clever repairs raised Truth, Justice, and the Constitution once more aloft—and *Calhoun* inspired South Carolina until the marble statesman lost his last debate in the fires of Columbia. (To imagine how Powers's *Calhoun* looked before its destruction, we nowadays must consult crude drawings or cruder reproductions. But since its head was based on a portrait bust by Powers that is still extant, we know that *Calhoun* was a splendid work of art: the sculptor had crossed neoclassicism with an American sense of the particular.)

Fuller has left us some of the most memorable essays, criticism, and journalism written by an American of her century. She was a Byron of our Romantic era, a Byron who rose above mere poetry. Fuller's best-known feminist passage, with a cruel irony, is the one in which she proposes that women ought to be sea captains, even. Her small son lies buried under a willowed monument to his mother in Mount Auburn Cemetery, flanked by the Emersons, Longfellows, Lowells, Hawthornes, and Holmeses with whom she was raised and with whom she belongs in her Transcendental heaven. Her epitaph reads, in part,

"BY BIRTH A CHILD OF NEW ENGLAND, BY ADOPTION A CITIZEN
OF ROME, BY GENIUS BELONGING TO THE WORLD."

Calhoun destroyed by fire and Fuller by water; South Carolina and Massachusetts; states-rights senator and meliorist
feminist—the space left by these two Americans is the air we
breathe today. A stern moralist might argue that a ship of state
with such cargo aboard would under any circumstances have
been doomed to shipwreck. Rougher ideas, principles more at
odds, rivalries more ancient have washed ashore since that day
off Fire Island. But the statues in our parks smeared with graffiti
tell only one part of our national story. The better part is told
by the stunning public art of a subsequent century which has
engaged an audience far wider than that of Powers, Greenough,
and Crawford. American masters of sculpture of this century
include Alexander Calder, David Smith, Richard Serra, Mark de
Suvero, Louise Nevelson, Claes Oldenburg, Richard Lippold,
and Richard Stankiewicz, for starters. Their melting-pot names
and works go far to realize the dream of Margaret Fuller that
"an original idea must animate this nation and fresh currents of
life must call into life fresh thoughts along its shores . . . that
day will not come until the fusions of the many races here is
accomplished [and] until moral and intellectual freedom are
prized as highly as political freedom."

5. MARGARET FULLER AND
THE DANCING SERPENT

A te voir marcher en cadence,
  Belle d'abandon,
On dirait un serpent qui danse
  Au bout d'un baton.

(To watch your rhythmic walk
  Beautiful and wild
Reminds one of a dancing snake
  At the tip of a rod.)

—Charles Baudelaire, "Le Serpent Qui Danse," 1857

Poets over the centuries have often compared women to snakes, but in the nineteenth century they carried the comparison to sinuous extremes. Among those serpentine extravaganzas, Baudelaire had two competitors from the medical field, John Keats and Oliver Wendell Holmes. The medical career of John Keats, surgical dresser at Guy's Hospital, was by no means as distinguished as that of Dr. Oliver Wendell Holmes, who by 1853 had become Parkman Professor of Anatomy and dean of the Harvard Medical School. On the other hand, Holmes was no Keats. Each wrote a work of caducean fantasy, but whereas Keats's long poem "Lamia" (1820) remains in the poetic canon, Holmes's "medicated" novel, *Elsie Venner* (1861), must be sought in the back wards of antiquarian bookdealers. That's a pity, if only because Margaret Fuller is far more engaging as Dr.

Holmes's title character than as Zenobia in Hawthorne's better-known *Blithedale Romance.*

Holmes puts his fanciful tale to moral use. He preaches the meliorist sermon that if human guilt lies in the gene—in nature rather than nurture, as it might be put now—then the guilty are more to be pitied than censured. Borrowing major elements from Keats's "Lamia," Holmes turns Elsie Venner into a fictional demon, half woman, half serpent. Like Lamia's, Elsie's magic is eclipsed by more powerful tricks of masculine science. But, for all those similarities, the judgment of literary history is probably correct: a modern reading of "Lamia" yields the heady thrill of glorious verse, while a study of *Elsie Venner* tells us that Margaret Fuller, his schoolmate, retained the fancy of Oliver Wendell Holmes forever.

The modern reader will appreciate not only the Freudian but also the genetic aspects of the woman-as-serpent theme. Who today does not carry in the mind's eye that serpentine image of DNA, a double helix on a central rod? How prescient of Baudelaire—unaware of DNA—to picture his Creole mistress as a dancing snake at the tip of a rod! It could, of course, be argued that the sinuous walk of Jeanne Duval might have raised reptilian thoughts in any random Parisian. But the poet has touched on an image from the most archaic regions of our cultural storehouse. Baudelaire's snake, *belle d'abandon* at the tip of a *baton*, is no simple stand-in for Freudian plumbing. From Eve to Apollo, Moses to Aesculapius, Hygeia to Hermes, the coiled serpent has guarded mystery, knowledge, and healing.

Doctors sport the caduceus of Hermes, twin snakes wound about a rod *en cadence*; scientists scan the twin coils of DNA wound on their central axis. What a concordance between the paraphernalia of an ancient art and the central structure of our new biology! The caduceus of Greek myth was Apollo's gift to Hermes in trade for a stolen lyre, and Hermes used his magic wand to cast spells, to transmute species, and to raise the dead.

These days, there is no end to the metamorphoses we can bring about with our wand of DNA.

The caduceus, winged at the top and entwined by serpents, is symbol of the power of Apollo and the magic of snakes. The pythons who guarded Apollo's temple were believed to share with their master the divine arts of prophecy and healing, of prognosis and therapeutics. Aesculapius appeared in the dreams of his patients as an undulant snake, while Hygeia was depicted with cup and adder. At the last *fin de siècle*, Gustav Klimt painted an erotic image of the goddess on the wall of the medical school in Vienna; the eyes of her snake stare out at the students. Athenian and Viennese may have looked at their fate in the eyes of ophidians, but *plus ça change*, as we say: a serpentine model of the double helix guards the entrance to my medical school, while in the courtroom life or death hangs on the evidence of DNA.

A suitable introduction to the woman-as-serpent theme is John Keats's "Lamia." The poem is not only Keats's meditation on the Lady Eve and metamorphosis but also an essay on the genetics of guilt. In "Lamia," Hermes chases a nymph over hill and dale in charming Crete. The nymph becomes lost and Hermes forlorn, but suddenly the messenger stumbles on

> . . . *a palpitating snake,*
> *Bright, and cirque couchant in a dusky brake.*
>
> *She was a gordian shape of dazzling hue,*
> *Vermilion-spotted, golden, green, and blue;*
> *Striped like a zebra, freckled like a pard,*
> *Eyed like a peacock, and all crimson barr'd; . . .*
> *Her head was serpent, but ah, bitter-sweet!*
> *She had a woman's mouth with all its pearls complete . . .*

This reptile charmer, whose unique aspect must be considered in the context of English dentistry, exacts a promise from

Hermes to transmute her form to human; in return, she will tell Hermes where his nymph is hidden. It all works as promised: the nymph is found, Hermes exults, and Lamia swoons. Fulfilling his part of the bargain, Hermes turns with snake-entwined wand

> *To the swoon'd serpent, and with languid arm,*
> *Delicate, put to proof the lythe Caducean charm . . .*
>
> *Left to herself, the serpent now began*
> *To change; her elfin blood in madness ran . . .*

What a Romantic precedent for the by-now-routine method of genetic manipulation known as homologous recombination! Our modern molecular biologists effect this sort of transformation at will; almost every human gene worth knowing has been spliced into other species. In Keats's poem, Lamia has been transformed into "a maid / More beautiful than ever twisted braid." But she is more than just a pretty transgenic face. Since she was constructed—in the words of molecular biologists—to retain and express on induction the serpentine genes of passion, she became:

> *A virgin purest lipp'd, yet in the lore*
> *Of love deep learned to the red heart's core:*
> *Not one hour old, yet of sciential brain*
> *To unperplex bliss from its neighbor pain . . .*
> *Intrigue with the specious chaos, and disport*
> *Its most ambiguous atoms with sure art; . . .*

Thus equipped, Lamia hies to Corinth, where she ensnares a young philosopher, Lycius. The two become enraptured with each other, enter an elaborate palace suddenly created for their tryst—she is after all a supernatural creature—and hold a wild, drunken prenuptial feast:

> *But when the happy vintage touch'd their brains*
> *Louder they talk, and louder come the strains*
> *Of powerful instruments:—the gorgeous dyes,*
> *The space, the splendor of the draperies,*
> *The roof of awful richness, nectarous cheer*
> *Beautiful slaves, and Lamia's self, appear . . .*

The Corinthian Eden contains more than one serpent. One of the wedding guests is Apollonius, a Sophist who has been Lycius' mentor, and this "bald-head Philosopher" immediately perceives that Lamia is a dangerous demon and fixes his knowing eyes directly on her. In his withering gaze, the beautiful creature cringes; she turns white and cold. Then, when Apollonius finally denounces her as a dangerous serpent, she vanishes into thin air. The old Sophist turns to his befuddled pupil:

> *Fool! Fool!*
> *. . . from every ill*
> *Of life have I preserv'd thee to this day,*
> *And shall I see thee made a serpent's prey?*

Lycius cannot bear this loss; he dies a languorous death of grief. In the last couplet of the poem his friends:

> *Supported him—no pulse, or breath they found,*
> *And, in its marriage robe, the heavy body wound.*

Lamia's story could be said to be a Romantic hint at Alfred North Whitehead's insight that the most heartrending aspect of science is the death of beautiful theory at the hands of ugly fact. Keats had it right. More often than not, it is the task of the bald-head professor to dash the fancies of the young on the rock of experience. One could argue that these dynamics of the family romance provide the energy that keeps both art and science moving.

Keats was at the center of the new medical science of his day. His teachers—Astley Cooper, William Babington, and Alexander Marcet—were respected scientists as well as physicians. As his letters tell us, Keats's feverish indecision between careers in the clinic and science, medicine and poetry, provided much of the energy behind "Lamia." Apollonius—no accidental name—is cast as the scientist/physician who, by Newtonian optics, has destroyed the beauty of the rainbow itself:

> . . . *Do not all charms fly*
> *At the mere touch of cold philosophy?*
> *There was an awful rainbow once in heaven:*
> *We know her woof, her texture; she is given*
> *In the dull catalogue of common things*
> *Philosophy will clip an Angel's wings . . .*
> *Unweave a rainbow, as it erewhile made*
> *The tender-person'd Lamia melt into a shade.*

One senses in this splendid passage the reason why Keats chose poetry, the Angel's wings, over his apothecary profession, over the "cold philosophy" of natural science.

When Holmes, who spent his life straddling the two callings, took up the challenge of "Lamia" a generation later, he turned the woman-as-serpent theme into an essay on Margaret Fuller and the genetics of gender. The critical fact of *Elsie Venner*—which we learn only after a warm-up account of what it means to be a Brahmin—is that the mother of strange and beautiful Elsie Venner has been bitten by a snake before Elsie was born. Elsie's "ophidian eyes and long neck" therefore become the external marks of a kink in her genes. No wonder she brings trouble to all she meets; no wonder she presides over Gothic and dark happenings!

As Holmes confided in letter and memoir, Elsie's serpentine features and ambiguous gender were patterned after Margaret Fuller, his classmate in the Cambridgeport school. Holmes described her as a nine-year-old schoolgirl with "a watery, aquamarine luster in her light eyes, and a long flexible neck, arching and undulating in strange sinuous movements." When he showed Margaret one of his compositions, she called it "trite," a word Holmes had never encountered. He was miffed at being bested by a girl. "I felt had drawn a prize, a five-dollar one at least, in the grand intellectual life lottery," Holmes wrote immodestly. He reckoned that Margaret must also be counted a winner, and he remained impressed. He dedicated his first book, *The Autocrat of the Breakfast Table*, to "The Schoolmistress," referring to Margaret Fuller's Providence days at the progressive Greene Street school.

When he came to write *Elsie Venner*, Holmes harked back to his school days. The fictional Elsie captivates her young schoolmaster, a student at the Harvard Medical School taking time out to teach. The very real Dr. Edwin Dickinson, a recent Harvard medical graduate who was also marking time, taught both Holmes and Fuller at the Cambridgeport school. A book of verse on Elsie's desk is open to Keats's "Lamia." Holmes had not only lectured extensively on Keats and "Lamia" but also knew that Keats's niece Emma had been Margaret Fuller's student and boarder in Providence. Keats's brother, George, who was in the United States to find his fortune, put Emma "under Fuller's wing" in 1837 while he disentangled himself from a messy business deal with John James Audubon on the Mississippi River. (The avian connection is curious here.)

All those elements—Keats and Lamia, Fuller and schoolrooms, serpents and medical students—are the ingredients of Holmes's Gothic novel. In *Elsie Venner*, Holmes introduces us to Elsie/Margaret as the young temptress:

> She narrowed her lids slightly, as one often sees a sleepy cat narrow hers,—somewhat as you may remember our famous Margaret used to, if you remember her at all,—so that her eyes looked very small, but bright as the diamonds on her

breast . . . the asp-like bracelet never left her arm. She was
never seen without some necklace,—either the golden cord
she wore at the great party, or a chain of mosaics, or simply
a ring of golden scales. The old Doctor felt very oddly as she
looked at him . . .

Elsie, we are told, owed her ophidian aspects to her constitution
rather than her will. Holmes, conflating Elsie, Fuller, and Lamia,
describes her effect on his hero, the young doctor-to-be who is
teaching at a girls' school in western Massachusetts. "In his
dreams he was pursued by the glare of cold glittering eyes,—
whether they were in the head of a woman or of a reptile he
could not always tell." Holmes had obviously not read Baudelaire, but the parallel is striking with:

> *Tes yeux, où rien ne se révèle*
> *De doux ni d'amer,*
> *Sont deux bijoux froids où se mêle*
> *L'or avec le fer.*
>
> *(Your eyes that reveal nothing*
> *Either bitter or sweet,*
> *Are two cold jewels which mix*
> *Gleams of gold with iron.)*

Troubled by the attraction of those cold glittering eyes and
by strange goings-on at the school, the young man writes back
to his Harvard professor:

She has marks of genius,—poetic or dramatic,—I hardly
know which. She read a passage from Keats' *Lamia* the other
day, in the schoolroom, in such a way that I declare to you
I thought some of the girls would faint or go into fits. She is
very graceful, you know, and they will have it that she can
twist herself into all sorts of shapes, or tie herself in a knot if
she wants to. There is not one of them that will look her in

the eyes. I pity the poor girl; but, Doctor, I do not love her.
I would risk my life for her, if it would do her any good, but
it would be in cold blood. If her hand touches mine, it is not
a thrill of passion I feel running through me, but a very different emotion. Oh, Doctor! there must be something in that
creature's blood which has killed the humanity in her.

Elsie Venner is a fictional construct in which nature and nurture are hybridized, much in the way we are now able to anneal
the Watson and Crick strands of DNA in the dish. Holmes gives
his professional opinion of the creature:

Here was a magnificent organization, superb in vigorous
womanhood, with a beauty such as never comes but after
generations of culture; yet through all this rich nature there
ran some alien current of influence, sinuous and dark, as when
a clouded streak seams the white marble of a perfect statue
. . . One [strain in her nature] made her a woman, with all a
woman's powers and longings. The other chilled all the currents of outlet for her emotions. It made her tearless and
mute, when another woman would have wept and pleaded.
And it infused into her soul something—it was cruel now to
call it malice—which was still and watchful and dangerous—
which waited its opportunity, and then shot like an arrow
from its bow out of the coil of brooding premeditation . . .
she was one of the creatures not to be tampered with,—silent
in anger and swift in vengeance.

A hybrid like this, from the back pages of the animal genome,
would have been polished off forthwith in detective stories by
Edgar Allan Poe, Arthur Conan Doyle, or even more virulent
social Darwinists such as Raymond Chandler. But Holmes, like
Keats, remains ever the good doctor; Holmes, like Keats, remains half in love with his half serpent. In his persona as the
Harvard professor, Holmes asks

the terrible question, how far the elements themselves are capable of perverting the moral nature: if valor, and justice, and truth, the strength of man and the virtue of woman, may not be poisoned out of a race by the food of the Australian in his forest,—the foul air and darkness of the Christians cooped up in the "tenement-houses" close by those who live in the palaces of the great cities?

The advice he offers the young student is a meliorist response to the question of good and evil. Holmes anticipates a very modern view not only of criminal justice but also of biochemical genetics:

> Treat bad men exactly as if they were insane . . . sit down and contemplate them charitably, remembering that nine tenths of their perversity comes from outside influences, drunken ancestors, abuse in childhood, bad company, from which you have happily been preserved, and for some of which you, as a member of society, may be fractionally responsible. I think also that there are *special influences* which *work in the blood like ferments.* [Holmes's italics]

Holmes clearly believed that a special influence working in Elsie Venner's blood like a ferment was the cause of Elsie's abnormal appearance and behavior. What a neat presentiment of the "one gene, one enzyme" hypothesis of molecular biology! Holmes's Gothic novel, which holds up surprisingly well on rereading, also addresses the ambiguities of gender, filled as it is with undertones of phallic serpents, forbidden wisdom, and barren wombs. But the author's half love for the pythoness turns Holmes's "medicated" novel into a very humane plea indeed. The professor pleads with us to remember that those for whom biology is destiny, like poor Elsie, or "our famous" Margaret— or Katharine Lee Bates for that matter—cannot change the hand they have been dealt. In fact and in fiction, their fate is directed

by constitution rather than will. In his novel, as from the bedside, Holmes asked no personal favor but begged to be "heard
in behalf of the women whose lives are at stake, until some
stronger voice shall plead for them."

✳

On October 16, 1845, a disheveled Edgar Allan Poe gave a poetry reading to a Lyceum audience in Boston. He had already
launched a series of polemics against the "transcendentalists,
Swedenborgians, abolitionists, and Harvard professors" who
dominated the New England literary scene. Poe had even gone
out of his way to call Margaret Fuller "a detestable old maid."
But that evening, facing the Brahmins, he was more confused
than combative. Thomas Wentworth Higginson noted that Poe,
"in a sort of persistent, querulous way, which . . . impressed me
at the time as nauseous flattery," went on to throw his audience
into sheer stupor. After an extensive apology for not having
delivered new material, Poe read in toto his early, befuddled
poem "Al Aaraaf." The audience dwindled rapidly, presumably
because, like Higginson, they were mystified and perplexed. Not
even an impromptu recital of "The Raven" could rescue the
evening. The occasion confirmed Lowell's final estimate:

> *There comes Poe, with his raven, like Barnaby Rudge,*
> *Three fifth of him genius and two fifth sheer fudge.*

The months after the debacle were followed by what Poe's
astute biographer, Kenneth Silverman, has called "the Lyceum
Wars." The unsparing Boston reviews of his Lyceum performance were answered by Poe with a torrent of invective, shotgun
critique, and *ad personam* attacks, most published in his own
Broadway Journal. He went out of his way to accuse the Boston
literati of cronyism, muddleheadedness, and plagiarism. Predict-
ably, Longfellow was the chief target. Poe then committed the
unforgivable: he spoke ill of Boston itself—its food, hotels, the

architecture of its state house, and the squalor of its duck pond, now invaded by frogs. Dr. Holmes eventually had the last word in *The Professor at the Breakfast Table*:

> After a man begins to attack the State House, when he gets bitter about the Frog-pond, you may be sure that there is not much left of him. Poor Edgar Poe died in the hospital soon after he got into this way of talking . . . Remember poor Edgar! He is dead and gone, but the State House has its cupola fresh-gilded, and the Frog-pond has got a fountain that squirts up a hundred feet into the air.

The plagiarism issue is amusing in this context. For Poe, who was an ex-West Pointer and ex-Virginian, his quarrel with the Boston literary establishment of reformers, abolitionists, and feminists was another aspect of his internal war between fact and fancy, science and art. Like Keats, he was drawn to many aspects of science and mathematics, but squelched them in favor of poetic urges. Poe's earliest book of verse, in 1829, contains this "Sonnet to Science":

> *Science! true daughter of Old Time thou art!*
> *Who alterest all things with thy peering eyes.*
> *Why preyest thou thus upon the poet's heart,*
> *Vulture, whose wings are dull realities?*
> *How should he love thee? or how deem thee wise,*
> *Who wouldst not leave him in his wandering*
> *To seek for treasure in the jewelled skies,*
> *Albeit he soared with an undaunted wing?*
> *Hast thou not dragged Diana from her car?*
> *And driven the Hamadryad from the wood*
> *To seek a shelter in some happier star?*
> *Hast thou not torn the Naiad from her flood,*
> *The Elfin from the green grass, and from me*
> *The summer dream beneath the tamarind tree?*

Silverman points out that Poe appropriated not only his "Diana from her car" but also "Hamadryad from the wood" and "Naiad from her flood," wood nymph and freshwater nymph, respectively, from an English translation of Jacques-Henri Bernardin de Saint Pierre's *Études de la Nature*. And "Lamia" is another source. We can spot that Keats's "the dull catalogue of common things" wound up as Poe's vulture whose "wings are dull realities." We can also read how Poe transformed Keats's line "Philosophy will clip an Angel's wings," turning Keats's general worry into a kind of personal affront: self-referent Poe "soared with an undaunted wing" until Philosophy clipped it, so to speak. After plagiarism charges were flying hot and heavy between Poe and the New England writers, Poe appended a footnote to the 1845 edition of his sonnet: "Private reasons— some of which have reference to the sin of plagiarism . . . have induced me, after some hesitation, to re-publish these, the crude compositions of my earliest boyhood.")

Poe's "Science" sonnet is not just a clumsy gloss on "Lamia" but also an introduction to the poet's many dark moods and black birds to come. The poem may also yield a clue to Poe's irate attacks on Longfellow, Lowell, Higginson, and the rest. In the antebellum period, the North in general, and Boston in particular, was regarded by Southerners as a rampart of Roundhead values, concerned with the "dull realities" of science, machines, and trade. Poe, on the other hand, fancied himself a son of the Cavalier South. A sometime soldier, disinherited but awash in plantation longings, he yearned on Broadway for the summer dream beneath the tamarind tree. No wonder that Charles Baudelaire, dreaming of the Indies on the Quai d'Anjou, worshiped Poe from afar and became his champion with the *hachischistes*.

These days, the North-South axis, the meridian between Boston and Richmond, between duty and languor, attracts at its southern extreme many writers who are disenchanted by modern science. Some are simply unlettered citizens of Peter Me-

dawar's "Pluto's Republic"; others adhere to the feel-good
tradition of the antinomians who believed, according to David
Hume, that the "obligations of natural law are suspended for
them." A model example of this modern antinomian fiction is
E. L. Doctorow's novella *The Waterworks* (1994), in which a
freelance writer and critic named Martin Pemberton serves as a
stand-in for Poe. The book is set in 1871, two decades after
Poe's death of alcoholism in Baltimore. Pemberton has disappeared from the streets of New York after a literary row with
Boston Brahmins. Pemberton's editor, the narrator of *The Waterworks*, receives a packet of journals which includes:

> the latest issue of that organ of Brahmin culture, the *Atlantic
> Monthly*, [with] an article by no less a personage than Oliver
> Wendell Holmes. Holmes was railing at certain ignorant New
> York critics who were not sufficiently in awe of his fellow
> trinomials of New England literary genius, James Russell
> Lowell, Henry Wadsworth Longfellow, and Thomas Went-
> worth Higginson. Though he didn't identify the offending
> critics, it was clear from his references that Martin Pemberton
> was one of them—I had run his piece on the subject early in
> the year, in which he had said of those men, and Mr. Holmes
> with them, that their names were too long for the work they
> produced.

The story continues as an antinomian version of a Poe tale in
which the obligations of natural law are artfully suspended:
Pemberton's father, a war profiteer, slave runner, and master of
a gloomy Hudson River mansion called Ravenswood, has been
long dead and buried, but Martin has seen him alive again and
carted about the city in a horse-drawn omnibus. Martin succeeds
in finding his father, who together with other aging capitalists
has been kept alive by a sinister physician-scientist named Dr.
Sartorius. Sartorius (tailor, or Schneider) is one of a distinguished line of medical threats to belletristic culture: Drs. Frank-

enstein, Moreau, Caligari, *und so weiter.* The good doctor is
keeping these senior citizens puffing around a sci-fi Xanadu hidden among the waterworks of the Croton reservoir. The old
boys have been rejuvenated by means of vital fluids and cells
extracted from the still-living bodies of abducted street orphans.
Martin himself becomes a captive of the evil doctor, and witnesses the exchange of youth for age:

> And what was this work, at least as I could fathom it? I saw
> him transfuse blood from one living being to another. I saw
> him with a hypodermic tube inject cellular matter into dead-
> ened brains. I saw first one, then another, of the orphan chil-
> dren begin to age, like leaves turning yellow . . . He drew
> their blood. I came to understand the pure scientific temper-
> ament as it shone from this man. It produced a mind that was
> unshockable, a man for whom there was no sacrilege . . .

A bit later the narrator confesses: "I could not sleep, I was
haunted . . . not by ghosts, but by Science. I felt afflicted with
intolerable reality." Poe, of course, was there first with his:
"Why preyest thou thus upon the poet's heart, / Vulture, whose
wings are dull realities?"

The new antinomians believe that the "intolerable reality" of
science is an aspect of a sinister world order, a world of fact
without value, a world ruled, as in *The Waterworks*, by "a
concordance of wealth, and government, and science . . ." The
narrator goes Poe one better in his overt iteration of the
haunted-by-science theme:

> Ever since this day I have dreamt sometimes . . . I, a street
> rat in my soul, dream even now . . . that if it were possible
> to lift this littered, paved Manhattan from the earth . . . A
> season or two of this and the mute, protesting culture buried
> for so many industrial years under the tenements and factories
> . . . would rise again . . . of the lean, religious Indians of the

bounteous earth, who lived without money or lasting architecture, flat and close to the ground—hunting, trapping, fishing, growing their corn and praying . . . always praying in
solemn thanksgiving for their clear and short life in this quiet
universe. Such love I have for those savage polytheists of my
mind . . . those friends of light and leaf.

Science, the Poe-folk tell us, gives us dreary fact and city litter;
only prayer and solemn thanksgiving will save us!

Dr. Oliver Wendell Holmes and his fellow Bostonians would
have found this revisionist fantasy of Indian life more than a
little disingenuous. "Thanksgiving for their clear and short life"?
Who would presume to tell *anyone* that early and violent death
of one's wife and children from infective disease is preferable to
survival? It has been estimated that the Native American population had a life expectancy of one generation. And as for those
clear and short lives spent "so many industrial years under the
tenements and factories," the actual numbers may be worth not-
ing. The death rate in New York City in 1845, that pre-tenement
and pre-industrial era of Edgar Allan Poe, was 27.3 per thousand
per year and the average life expectancy was in the forties. In
our day, New York City's death rate has dropped to 9.1 per
1,000 and our life expectancy risen to almost eighty. That was
no achievement of street rats or nostalgic literati but of trinomials such as Dr. Holmes and other sanitarians—among them
Frederick Law Olmsted and George Templeton Strong—who
washed their hands, cleaned the waters, built our sewers, and
dried the swamps.

The landscape of science has its own horizons, and they are
at least as wide as those of the "savage polytheists . . . those
friends of light and leaf." A photograph in the Harvard Medical
School archives shows a reflective Dr. Holmes in his library; he
is by no means either hunting, trapping, fishing—or growing his
corn and praying. He is surrounded by high bookshelves filled
with ancient and modern volumes of poetry, history, romance,

anatomy, histology, and pathology. Holmes has looked up from his microscope and appears to be puzzling out something new that he has just found under the lens. Although he is more than sixty years old in the photo, he retains that look of the perpetually young caught by Katharine Lee Bates in "The Library":

> *Visions shall come and go*
> *On the dreaming eyes of youth,*
> *And here shall her chosen know*
> *The countenance of truth.*

The complex human side of a nature like Holmes's—with its nose for cant, ear for verse, and eye for the new—guaranteed his countrymen that the century of science would not spell the end of the imagination. Holmes and his fellow trinomials— James Russell Lowell, Henry Wadsworth Longfellow, and Thomas Wentworth Higginson—would not have been haunted by the science of our day. They would have been pleased that we have acquired the power to refigure the strands of our own DNA, to twirl in any direction those twin serpents at the tip of our baton. No antinomian himself, Ralph Waldo Emerson looked forward to the day when scientists would be able to "make an animalcule incontestably swimming and jumping before my eyes. I should only feel that it indicated that the day had arrived when the human race might be trusted with a new degree of power, and its immense responsibility; for these steps [are] only a hint of an advanced frontier supported by an advancing race behind it."

6. EMERSON, AGASSIZ, AND THE SUBMARINE CABLE

Thoreau and Hawthorne excepted, the men and women of the American Renaissance were convinced that mass communication would expand the national spirit: lead type and the Morse code were tools in the workshop of democracy, they believed. The coiled transatlantic cable became a dominant image of American progress for them, much in the way that the double helix of DNA has served our century. In his journal poem "The Adirondacs," Emerson describes how in August 1858 he heard:

> . . . Of the wire-cable laid beneath the sea,
> And landed on our coast, and pulsating
> With ductile fire. Loud, exulting cries
> From boat to boat, and to the echoes round,
> Greet the glad miracle. Thought's new-found path
> Shall supplement henceforth all trodden ways,
> Match God's equator with a zone of art,
> And lift man's public action to a height
> Worthy the enormous cloud of witnesses.

Emerson was embarked on an Adirondack canoe expedition when the news came of this first submarine cable link between the continents. He and his colleagues—ten gentlemen and scholars from Boston—had been corralled by the artist-diplomat William J. Stillman to make a pilgrimage to the virgin lakes and forests of the Adirondacks. The expedition included not only

Emerson, the young country's leading moral philosopher, but also Louis Agassiz, its major natural philosopher. They were joined by, among others, Dr. Jeffries Wyman, an eminent anatomist; James Russell Lowell of *The Atlantic Monthly*; and Dr. Oliver Wendell Holmes's brother John. They "swept with oars the Saranac," endured "Hard fare, hard bed and comic misery —the midge, the blue-fly and mosquito," but, thrilled over the pure Alpine element they breathed, they "trode on air."

Under canvas in what was called "the Philosopher's Camp," each Boston nabob did what he did best. Lowell shot at an osprey and climbed a tree. Emerson sniffed pine and wrote verse. Agassiz was the one most completely in his element. With Wyman as assistant, he "dissected the slain deer, weighed the trout's brain," captured "lizard, salamander, shrew crab, mice, snail, dragon-fly, minnow and moth." Those exercises were followed by a hearty meal of venison, beans, trout, and ale. Agassiz regaled them with stories of his student days with Baron Cuvier in Paris, his theories of glaciers and the ice age, and the mating habits of European fish. It is difficult to understand why bluff Jean Louis Rodolphe Agassiz (1802–73), whose legacy to modern science is dubious, was so highly treasured by the lettered folk of his time. Lowell, Holmes, Wyman, and Emerson—indeed all the lights of Boston—were in awe of this Swiss polymath. But if we measure his works against those of the grand system builders of Europe—Linnaeus, Buffon, Lamarck, Cuvier, Lyell, Darwin—or look into the accounts of his shady business ventures, it becomes easier to understand why he left Switzerland for fame and fortune in the New World.

Having left his first wife to die of tuberculosis in Europe, Agassiz insinuated himself into the Brahmin aristocracy. Indeed, his second wife, Elizabeth Cabot Cary Agassiz, was to become the first president of Radcliffe, and *her* paternal grandfather was Colonel Thomas H. Perkins, the benefactor who established the Perkins Institution for the "Grecian and blind-compelling" Dr. Samuel Gridley Howe. (The appointment of Agassiz as professor of zoology at Harvard in 1847 must have pleased his sister-in-law, Mary Louisa Cary, who happened to be the wife of the professor of Greek and future president of Harvard College, Cornelius Felton. The Carys and Perkinses were childhood playmates of Horace Greenough—and he of course was the brother-in-law of Julia Ward Howe!) With backers of this sort, Agassiz went into the lucrative but risky business of peddling his folios of natural history à la John James Audubon. In the process he became involved in a series of drawn-out lawsuits with publishers, colleagues, and employees. He was also a complete and contentious denier of Darwinian evolution, a didact of prodigious energy, and the model of professorial disdain. Nevertheless, he managed to find time to father marine biology in America.

In the New World as in the Old, Agassiz established his reputation as a master taxonomist, collector, and naturalist; he was by no means a master citizen of our young republic. This Barnum of Biology knew little and cared less about American politics and found the problem of slavery nothing but a distraction. It may be racing ahead of our chronology with respect to his 1858 trip with Emerson to the Adirondacks, but we should note that it took the Civil War to make his colleagues realize how hugely self-absorbed their Agassiz was. Agassiz had already been sufficiently "inconvenienced" by the revolutionary stirrings of 1830 in France and Switzerland and cited them as one of the reasons for his disaffection from Europe. He was therefore not about to be disturbed by such minor diversions from science as the Civil War. His student Edward Sylvester Morse describes the professor's reactions to Fort Sumter:

April 15, Monday: Intensely exciting news this morning. All the previous news confirmed. Lincoln calls for 75,000 men. Saturday Prof [Agassiz] after lecture told us what we should do. That we must work and show the people that amid such exciting times we should not go wild with the general excite-

ment but work. That we should not read the papers, etc. This
morning Ordway was reading a paper and Prof said we must
remember what he said on Saturday, and then went out of
the room. He immediately came back and said if we did not
think as he did, he should forbid every paper from coming
into the building.

Agassiz occupied his time during the war by amassing the
major biological collection that became Harvard's Museum of
Comparative Zoology. His wartime correspondence was devoted entirely to squeezing funds from the federal purse for the
purpose of collecting specimens; he also found time to explain
to Dr. Howe that the coloreds were genetically inferior, that
mulattos were sure to prove sterile, and that amalgamation of
the races was biologically unsound.

Putting the distractions of the Civil War behind him as soon
as possible, he resumed his elaborate, and remarkably well-
funded, collecting expeditions. In 1865 he trekked to South
America in search of specimens for his volume *Fishes of the New
World*. The expedition turned out to be an important one for
American science and letters, but not because of the fishes. On
that trip, young William James, who had signed on as one of
Agassiz's assistants, decided that fieldwork was not for him. Sea-
sick, bug-ridden, and feverish with the pox in Rio de Janeiro,
he wrote home: "No one has the right to write about 'The Nature of Evil' [the title of a book written by his father] or have
any opinion of evil who has not been at sea." Giving up taxonomy in the tropics, he proceeded via the Harvard Medical
School and a *Wanderjahr* in Germany to launch the modern
study of the mind.

Natural history, according to Agassiz, had no room for Darwin; he told his students that the study of nature was the study
of God. Agassiz, the natural philosopher, was more rigidly convinced than Emerson, the moral philosopher, that the purpose
of God was benign and could be read in the facts of nature.

"Study Nature, Not Books" reads the motto of Agassiz, now preserved in the library of the Marine Biological Laboratory at Woods Hole. "Study Books, You'll Learn More" the modern embryologist Eugene Bell has countered. He may have something there; of the two, Emerson was the great reader.

When Agassiz urged the study of nature rather than books, he was by no means encouraging his students to experiment *with* nature; that was left for the Claude Bernards of physiology and the William Jameses of psychology. One could say that Agassiz believed that the task of the naturalist is to marvel, to number, to name, and then to marvel once again. The irony is that although in his lifetime Agassiz was as well known by educated folk as were Emerson, Lowell, and Longfellow, he is nowadays chiefly remembered, even by biologists, for that call to the lab at Woods Hole. He is also remembered by doctors of a certain age who were exposed to Dr. Holmes's poem on the technique of physical examination:

> Don't clutch his carpus in your icy fist,
> But warm your fingers ere you take the wrist.
> If the poor victim needs must be percussed,
> Don't make an anvil of his aching bust,
> (Doctors exist within a hundred miles
> Who thump a thorax as they'd hammer piles;)
> If you must listen to his doubtful chest,
> Catch the essentials, and ignore the rest . . .
> So of your questions; don't in mercy try
> To pump your patient absolutely dry;
> He's not a mollusk, squirming in a dish
> You're not Agassiz, and he's not a fish.

On the day the sages of the Philosopher's Camp crossed Tupper Lake they were shown a newspaper which carried news of the completion of the transatlantic cable. Emerson was energized by the possibility of communication between the continents. He imagined that it might someday be feasible to use electrical impulses to mimic—or to substitute for—the machinery of human mentation. Electricity for Emerson was:

> *A spasm throbbing through the pedestals*
> *Of Alp and Andes, isle and continent,*
> *Urging astonished Chaos with a thrill*
> *To be a brain, or serve the brain of man.*

But even the Adirondacks, that arcadia of lake and mountain, that paradise of fish and philosopher, contained the serpent of doubt. *Et in Arcadia Ego!* One or another of the academics—most had Harvard appointments—was miffed that this technical triumph of the age had been brought about by businessmen, and not professors; commerce and not natural philosophy had won the prize. But, unlike his professional companions, Emerson was not troubled that:

> *. . . a hungry company*
> *Of traders, led by corporate sons of trade,*
> *perversely borrowing from the shop the tools*
> *Of science, not from the philosophers,*
> *Had won the brightest laurel of all time.*

Emerson, Transcendentalism forsworn, argued that it mattered not whether this achievement was the result of pure or applied science; there was glory enough for all. For all, indeed, except the subject races:

> *It is not Iroquois or cannibals,*
> *But ever the free race with the front sublime,*
> *And these instructed by their wisest too,*
> *Who do the feat, and lift humanity.*

Emerson believed that transatlantic communication would bring to everyone in the New World—paleface, redskin, black man—the noble vision of the wider, albeit Western, culture. There was also no doubt in his mind that ordinary folk would benefit from instruction by the wisest. Nor did he doubt that the sages of Boston would be there to help lift humanity to its feat, as it were. He hoped that the cultural desert of the New World would become transformed by its newfound means of communication with the Old:

> *What in the desert was impossible*
> *Within four walls is possible again,—*
> *Culture and libraries, mysteries of skill,*
> *Traditioned fame of masters, eager strife*
> *Of keen competing youths, joined or alone*
> *To outdo each other and extort applause.*
> *Mind wakes a new-born giant from her sleep.*
> *Twirl the old wheels! Time takes fresh start again,*
> *On for a thousand years of genius more.*

The poem is such a sanguine tribute to the energy of an industrial, scientific age that one barely believes the poet who wrote "Brahma" could have written it. Nor does it sound like the Transcendental Emerson of *The Dial*. No, "Twirl the old wheels! Time takes fresh start again" sounds almost like Whitman, as well it might. Whitman had also called for the new:

> *Unscrew the locks from the doors!*
> *Unscrew the doors themselves from their jambs!*

Three years earlier, Whitman had sent a copy of his *Leaves of Grass* to Emerson, whom he idolized. Emerson wished him joy of his "free and brave thought. I greet you at the beginning of a great career, which yet must have had a great foreground for such a start." The influences seemed to flow in both direc-

tions. Whitman was no less sanguine about science than any
Brahmin:

Hurrah for positive science! Long live exact demonstration!
Fetch stonecrop and mix with cedar and branches of lilac;
This is the lexicographer or chemist . . . this made a grammar of
   old cartouches
These mariners put the ship through dangerous unknown seas
This is the geologist and this works with the scalpel . . .

As was his wont, James Russell Lowell struck a loftier tone
when he returned from that canoe trip to the Adirondacks. His
homage to the transatlantic cable, "Science and Poetry," is re-
lentlessly classical in allusion:

The Age of Wonder is renewed again,
And to our disenchanted day restores
The Shoes of Swiftness that give odds to Thought,
The Cloak that makes invisible; and with these
I glide, an airy fire, from shore to shore,
Or from my Cambridge whisper to Cathay.

Dr. Holmes, writing doggerel for his fellow Harvard alumni,
suggested that Yankee science could now rival even the French
—who had that unfair head start of the Enlightenment. Antic-
ipating much of the neurologic jargon of modern telecommu-
nication, which speaks of branches and nodes, networks and
nerve centers, Holmes compared the submarine cable to the planet's informational "spinal cord":

We've tried reform—and chloroform—and both have turned our
brain;
When France called up the photograph, we roused the foe to pain;
Just so those earlier sages shared the chaplet of renown,—
Hers sent a bladder to the clouds, ours brought their lightning
down . . .

We've seen the sparks of Empire fly beyond the mountain bars,
Till, glittering o'er the Western wave, they joined the setting stars;
And ocean trodden into paths that trampling giants ford.
To find the planet's vertebra and sink its spinal cord

These responses to nineteenth-century science express the rosiest of social sentiments. Emerson's electric future, where "culture and libraries, mysteries of skill" will come alive within four walls, is a dream of democratic enlightenment. Lowell's hymn to the airwaves predicts good odds on the swift diffusion of useful thought. Holmes's boast that Yankee know-how "roused the foe to pain"—anesthesia—is a direct link between democracy and discovery, "reform and chloroform." What a cheerful noise these poems make! Emerson twirls the old wheels, Whitman tears the doors from their jambs; he will go on to sing of the body electric. But, while these paeans to science differ widely in quality—Whitman is as grand as ever while Holmes is here very slight—the verses share a spirited music. The lines are alive with the sound of invention, a pulse of the new, an electric hum that today has become the most public of noises within four walls: the sound of America on-line.

Emerson, who joined to Transcendentalism a very Yankee respect for technology, listed in his journals the proudest achievements of his age. "In my lifetime have been wrought five miracles," he wrote, "namely, 1, the Steamboat; 2, the Railroad; 3, the Electric Telegraph; 4, the application of the Spectroscope to astronomy; 5, the Photograph;—five miracles which have altered the relations of nations to each other. Add cheap postage; and the mowing machine and the horse-rake." This passage, so much in keeping with his Adirondack tribute to the transatlantic cable, has been read by some as a shallow lampoon of American optimism. But one could also argue that Emerson's list forms the direct connection between the Flowering of New England and the Flowering of DNA. The men of the American Renaissance believed that there was a moral aspect to material progress;

they were convinced that science, pure or applied, would inevitably promote the public good over private gain. That Yankee belief links "cheap postage; and the mowing machine and the horse-rake" to the five miracles of invention. Emerson, as meliorist, was convinced that the spectroscope *and* the horse-rake, the telegraph *and* cheap postage, would raise our public acts to heights where angels soar:

> Greet the glad miracle. Thought's new-found path
> Shall supplement henceforth all trodden ways,
> Match God's equator with a zone of art,
> And lift man's public action to a height
> Worthy the enormous cloud of witnesses,
> When linked hemispheres attest his deed.

These days, Watson and Crick are said to bring us news far less reassuring than Emerson. Indeed, the determinists of genes, those fans of bell-shaped curves and the students of insect altruism, sound much more like Agassiz than Emerson. The gloomy tomes of sociobiology tell us that those double coils of DNA, those transatlantic strands now technically called "Watson" and "Crick" strands, have after all only one purpose: that of relentless, meaningless doubling. "It has not escaped our notice that this structure immediately suggests a copying mechanism" are not only the actual words of the Watson-Crick paper in *Nature* but also a blueprint for what Richard Dawkins has called *The Selfish Gene.* In its most reductive form, the new message of DNA is not that we are a little lower than the angels, but a little sloppier than a virus. For some of us, this is refreshing news indeed. Absolved of the need to divine the motive of its maker, we can begin to tinker with those runs of DNA, to meliorate its errors in the dish, and—in the Emersonian sense— make this "new-found path supplement henceforth the trodden paths" of crippling and disease.

Not long ago, I checked out Emerson's prophecies on Time-

Warner cable television. For is not our cable television system simply a fancier version of the submarine cable? How close have we come today to

> *Urging astonished Chaos with a thrill*
> *To be a brain, or serve the brain of man?*

On my local cable television system, the trial of O. J. Simpson was on two channels. In the middle of DNA evidence presented by the prosecution to show that Simpson was at the scene of the crime, the polymerase chain reaction was the subject of intense litigation; no big news there. ZAP! It also seemed to be Madonna's week. One could find the singer on no fewer than three channels at the same time. ZAP! On MTV, Madonna was shown as a defrocked nun. She sang to music not modal but tribal and, with rosary and crucifix as props, took the sort of anguished swipes at her body one might expect of a contortionist with hives. ZAP! On another channel she was dressed in stiff shards of black leather connected by enough belting, metal chains, and hobnailed bracelets to satisfy the needs for bondage of the Marquis de Sade himself. Flanked by six other similarly cachectic specters of uncertain gender, she crooned lyrics which sounded like a coyote's version of the Eton boating song. To paraphrase Yeats, it was difficult to tell the singer from the thong. ZAP! Now she was dressed like the Tin Man in *The Wizard of Oz*: twin metal funnels formed her poitrine. ZAP! ZAP!

But I was also connected to another world. ZAP! There was the late Leonard Bernstein leading the Berlin Philharmonic through Beethoven's Ninth Symphony; the chorus had reached Schiller's "Ode to Joy": *Traditioned fame of masters.* ZAP! Here was a distinguished cardiologist from Duke University describing the seven membrane-spanning segments of the beta-adrenergic receptor: *Mysteries of skill.* ZAP! Three graceful giraffes in uniforms of the Big Ten were in violent collision under a basketball hoop in a replay of the Final Four: *Eager strife of keen competing youths.* ZAP! There was Jacques Cousteau, our Agassiz of the airwaves, explaining the teleology of love among the manatees: *Twirl the old wheels!* ZAP! On another replay, that of the fortieth anniversary of the discovery of DNA, an aging Watson and Crick were looking at their makeshift model of the double helix. Crick had two palms outstretched as if to show stigmata. Look, he seemed to be saying, I'm St. Francis of the Cavendish: *Time takes fresh start again.* ZAP!

It could be argued from this evidence that Emerson's happy vision of the cable will not be denied. Despite the cackle of shysters or bleat of strumpets, the sounds pullulating on all those branches of the cable are voices of a democracy richer by far than the philosophers' cozy camp in the wilderness. The airwaves yield an electrical signal abuzz with the rich codes of life, perhaps well "worthy the enormous cloud of witnesses." Emerson had it right, for better or worse, whether the code be Morse or genetic. "Thought's new-found path shall supplement henceforth all trodden ways." Democracy and DNA.

II. WAR AND PEACE

Be that the glory of the past,
  With these our sacred toils begin:
So flies in tatters from its mast
  The yellow flag of sloth and sin,

And lo! the starry folds reveal
  The blazoned truth we hold so dear:
To guard is better than to heal
  The shield is nobler than the spear.

—Oliver Wendell Holmes,
  "For a Meeting of the National Sanitary Association," 1860

7. THE SANITARIANS OF CENTRAL PARK

In his account of a nerve-racking trip to Antietam, "My Hunt for the Captain" (1862), Dr. Holmes gave an early description of New York's Central Park, then only three years old and as yet incomplete:

> The Central Park is an expanse of wild country, well crumpled so as to form ridges which will give views and hollows that hold water. The hips and elbows and other bones of nature stick out here and there in the shape of rocks which give character to the scenery, and an unchangeable, unpurchasable look to a landscape that without them would have been in danger of being fattened by art and money out of all its native features. The roads were fine, the sheets of water beautiful, the bridges handsome, the swans elegant in their deportment, the grass green and as short as a fast horse's winter coat.

The doctor penned these sentiments while breaking his wartime journey in New York en route home from the battlefield with his son, Oliver Wendell Holmes, Jr. The father had recovered his gravely wounded son and was bringing him to Boston from the bloodiest day of battle ever fought on this continent. The Union's quasi-victory at Antietam permitted President Lincoln to announce the Emancipation Proclamation, an act which marked the progression of Northern war aims from a simple fight to save the Union to the more complex goal of abolishing slavery.

Historians tell us that the abolitionist spirit which culminated in the Proclamation was an expression of the Puritan charge to do God's work on earth. It was also the driving force behind the U.S. Sanitary Commission. It is therefore no accident that its executive secretary was the abolitionist, journalist, and self-trained landscape architect Frederick Law Olmsted of Hartford, Connecticut. Perhaps Olmsted's greatest architectural achievement was his plan for the Central Park of Manhattan which he and Calvin Vaux drafted in 1856. Certainly his most successful journalistic accomplishment was his book *The Cotton Kingdom*, an exposé of slavery's impact on Southern life. The Connecticut Yankee had made several long field trips to the rural South on behalf of *The New York Times* between 1853 and 1854 and concluded that "slavery not only degrades the slaves but demoralizes the masters and prevents agricultural progress." These reports, collected in *The Cotton Kingdom*, became important arguments in the service of abolition. Olmsted pointed out that ninety-nine of a hundred free workingmen of the North were fed four times better than the average hardest-worked slave on the Louisiana sugar plantations. Those slaves were worked with much greater severity than free laborers of the North. "On no farm, and in no factory, or mine, even when double wages are paid for night-work, did I ever hear of men or women working regularly eighteen hours a day." He went on to detail the squalor of life in Southern backwaters and the lack of culture in Southern cities—no singing societies, theaters, libraries, newspapers, publishers. "The people have almost no interest in literature or art, science or foreign affairs" except those which affected the price of cotton.

Olmsted's harshest critique was of Southern sanitary practices:

In my last journey of nearly three months between the Mississippi and the Upper James River . . . nine times out of ten, I slept in a room with others, in a bed which stank, supplied with but one sheet, if with any; I washed with utensils common to the whole household; I found no garden, no flowers, no fruit, no tea, no cream . . . no curtains, no lifting windows (three times out of four absolutely no windows), no couch— if one reclined in the family room it was on the bare floor— for there were no carpets or mats. For all that the house crawled with vermin.

Olmsted returned to New York a convert to the abolitionist cause. He had gone to the South convinced that a race he thought inferior would become "elevated" by steady contact with the more enterprising one. What he saw persuaded him that the backwardness of the South was regional and endemic, and that slavery was a transmissible disease which bred inefficiency in both slave and master. If slavery persisted, no "improvement" of science or art might be expected from either side of the lash. In that sense, he was of one mind with Holmes, who had written to his fellow Yankee John Lothrop Motley: "We are the conquerors of Nature, they of Nature's weaker children."

Morals and hygiene were permanently linked in the Yankee character, and therefore Olmsted's Central Park can be read as an architectural *summa* of two nineteenth-century reform movements: abolition and sanitation. How fitting, therefore, that they are commemorated by the two most notable statues in the park's precinct. Augustus Saint-Gaudens's equestrian figure of General William Tecumseh Sherman (1899) presides over the plaza at the southeastern corner of Central Park, while Florence Stebbins's *Angel of the Waters* (1862) tops the Bethesda Fountain at its center. The imposing gilt general, preceded by Victory, sports a cloak and a sword; the Angel, lily in hand, shades the fount with her hovering wings. They celebrate Justice militant and Healing sublime, or reform and chloroform, as Holmes had it.

In no small measure, the park was built in response to the cholera epidemics of 1848–49; its construction was a major issue of the 1850 mayoral campaign. Cholera had arrived in full force in the spring of 1849, following a year of revolution and large-scale emigration from Europe. The authorities in New York appropriated $55,000, vowing to "give our city a cleaning as it has not had in years." But despite strict quarantine, inspections of new immigrants at the port, and a great bout of street scrubbing, the summer of 1849 brought 18,000 cases of cholera and 8,000 deaths in a city of half a million inhabitants. And despite a national day of fasting and prayer declared by President Zachary Taylor at the high-water mark of the epidemic, cholera killed 1,178 New Yorkers on August 11, 1849.

Not until winter did the epidemic abate, and by then clean water and open spaces had become a political issue. It was clear that land free of "squatters, pigs and shanties" was needed. The cost of Central Park was staggering at the time—$5.5 million for the land alone. But proponents for the park argued that it was a price worth paying. Uncontaminated land was needed on which to place the reservoirs while the Croton water aqueducts were slowly put in service. But there was more to the park than water. The local commissioners charged with construction of Central Park hoped that this "barren waste might be converted into a good healthy pair of lungs for the entire population of the most enterprising City in the World." They were echoing Olmsted's conviction that there was a moral aspect to light and air and leisure, that a crowded, overworked city was prey to social as well as physical ills. In the interests of their white revolution, Olmsted and the sanitarians joined in a national political movement against dirt and disease, against rural sloth and urban squalor. A president of the National Sanitary Convention proclaimed in 1859, "Let the land be covered with sanitary associations and it will soon stand as much a landmark for the health, happiness and comfort of its people, as it is now a beacon light for the politically oppressed of other lands."

In the event, when cholera struck again at the end of the Civil War, in 1866, the park had been largely completed. *The New York Times* for August 19, 1866, lists the bills of mortality for cholera, then raging in the city. However, in the immediately adjacent column, its editors proudly note that Mr. Olmsted's Central Park is ready for summer recreation, having been won from "a dreary waste of sterile rocks, rising boldly and defiantly in the face of thrift and enterprise, relieved now and then by filthy sink-holes and pools of stagnant water . . . an excrescence on the fair features of the city." Only somewhat delayed by the war, the main conduits of the water supply were essentially connected; the reservoirs had been established, the aqueduct was flowing. The city was therefore ready to respond to cholera when the Sanitary Commission under George Templeton Strong decreed, "Sanitation, not quarantine is the answer!" He was correct, but when a cholera alert was sounded in April of that year, the city used both approaches, quarantine *and* sanitation.

The experience of Civil War contagion had permitted the U.S. Army Medical Department to reason that cholera and other intestinal diseases were in some fashion connected to contaminated water. New York appealed to Washington for help, and General of the Armies Ulysses S. Grant sent the "best man in the United States for the place." He was Dr. Edward Dalton, a Boston Brahmin who had been chief medical officer of the Army of the Potomac and in charge of the enormous base hospital at City Point, Virginia, which had served as many as ten thousand sick and wounded Union soldiers. Shortly after helping to clean up New York, Dalton was to die of ailments contracted at City Point. (For this reason, and for his work in battlefield surgery, Dalton is honored, alongside the two Lowell brothers and Robert Gould Shaw, as one of heroes to whom Soldiers' Field at Harvard is dedicated.)

The newly appointed Board of Health of New York designated Dalton as Sanitary Commissioner and granted him unusual authority. Despite complaints that his work had "been repeatedly obstructed by the interference of the Courts," his vigorous efforts paid off. Sixty subdistricts were established, in which public-health officers were detailed to search out and examine all new cases. More than 15,000 cellar dwellers were displaced from crowded tenements and housed in clean dormitories. Suspected cholera victims were trundled off to temporary hospitals on land and to new floating hospitals in the harbor. Crumbling water pipes were repaired, new sewers were dug, and reservoirs were strictly policed. Finally, Dalton established a disinfectant depot and laboratory at 308 Mulberry Street to support the disinfectant squads that scoured the city twenty-four hours a day. Their task was to clean and disinfect all premises where cholera cases had been reported and to apply disinfectants to the bodies of all cholera victims. As a result, although New York had grown to a population of 750,000 when the 1866 epidemic struck, only 1,200 of its citizens contracted cholera and only 600 died.

In war and peace, battlefield and city slum, Dalton, Strong, and the sanitarians proved Holmes's dictum: "The bills of mortality are more obviously affected by drainage than by this or that method of practice." And while cholera raged unchecked in other cities, *The New York Times* was able to boast in August 1866 that "Central Park to-day is an institution of which the nation may feel proud . . . take all day to stroll about at your leisure as we did. If you come away dissatisfied with the manner in which the Commissioners have expended the $4,829,016 placed at their disposal since the work was commenced, you will be the only individual out of the 7,593,139 persons who visited the Park who expresses one single word of complaint." Holmes was one of those, moaning that Mr. Olmsted's "remote pleasure ground" was a four-dollar hackney ride beyond the Pillars of Hercules of the fashionable quarter. He called it New York's *Ex*centric Park. But when Dr. Holmes visited it, Central Park was no longer Mr. Olmsted's pleasure ground. Olmsted was already in Washington with the Sanitary Commission. In his own fashion, he was fighting the good fight to bring down the Cotton Kingdom.

*

The U.S. Sanitary Commission was an independent association of reformist doctors, educated laymen, and ardent theologians who gathered in Washington for the express purpose of keeping the white revolution allied to the Union cause. Their meliorist ranks united abolitionist with Free-Soiler, Boston Brahmin with New York merchant, Transcendentalist with Quaker, homeopath with allopath, doctor with poet. Shortly after the fall of Fort Sumter, the sanitarians began their war efforts by offering medical assistance to the Union troops, and by war's end they had literally written the book on military hygiene, urban epidemics, and a safe water supply. Nowadays the work of the Sanitary Commission survives in venues other than Central Park. It is responsible for the sanitary ordinances we obey, the spaces we roam, the water we drink and—uniquely—for one hymn written on its stationery.

One year before Holmes visited Central Park, and after the Union debacle at Bull Run, Julia Ward Howe was unable to fall asleep in her Washington hotel room. She had come to the capital with her husband, Dr. Samuel Gridley Howe, to attend a meeting of the Sanitary Commission called by Olmsted. A melody that the dispirited Union soldiers had sung throughout the day kept repeating itself: "John Brown's body lies a-moldering in the grave." Perhaps because the Howes had founded the abolitionist Free Soil Party, perhaps because they had raised money for John Brown himself and had warmly received him at their home Green Peace, Mrs. Howe could not rid her mind of the John Brown melody. Troubled, she sat down at a table, and through the night, using the nearest stationery at hand, wrote out "The Battle Hymn of the Republic." She finished her poem as dawn rose over Washington. In the upper left-hand corner of the original manuscript is the guarantee of its origin:

Sanitary Commission, Washington, D.C.
Treasury Building   *Nov* 18 *61*

Shortly thereafter the hymn was published in Lowell's *Atlantic Monthly* and became almost overnight the anthem of abolition. After Antietam, it became in fact as in title the battle hymn of the Grand Army of the Republic. The lyrics "As Christ died to make men holy / Let us fight to make them free" could also serve as an epitaph for the Howes, who stood out among the ranks of abolitionists and sanitarians by virtue of their energy, courage, compassion—and wealth.

Julia Ward Howe was the daughter of Samuel Ward, a prominent New York merchant, banker, and patron of the arts. Thomas Cole painted his famous *The Voyage of Life* panels for the Wards, and those immensely popular paintings hung in the Wards' private picture gallery. Her brother, also Samuel Ward, married an Astor and became one of the founders of *The Nation* and of the New York Philharmonic.

Julia Ward found the perfect match in Samuel Gridley Howe. Dr. Howe, a Harvard Medical School product, was more than an effective advocate for the blind. A true social radical, he was an abolitionist who risked his life with what Thomas Wentworth Higginson described as a "constitutional love for freedom and for daring enterprises, taking more interest in action than in mere agitation." The actions he took were on behalf of Greek vs. Turk, Pole vs. Russian, Irish immigrant vs. Boston ruffian, fugitive slave vs. slave owner, abolitionist vs. Unionist—and finally North against South. He was also persuaded that dirt and disease were social ills. His idea of a medical career was, literally, a life in the trenches. He never failed to join the issue of medical care with that of freedom in general. From the field with the Sanitary Commission in 1861 he wrote:

Our soldiers in the Army of the Potomac are dying at the rate of three and a half in a hundred yearly; and in the Army of the West at the rate of five in a hundred . . . twenty-seven whole regiments laid low in a year, not by the sword, but by disease! Merciful Heaven! it almost drives one mad, when with this fearful fact before his eyes . . . pardon this outburst; but I lose patience at the delay to strike a righteous and killing blow into the very stomach of the rebellion by proclaiming emancipation under the war power, and enforcing it as fast and as far as we can; since every week's delay costs five hundred lives, and every month's two thousand . . . The Athenians rejected a plan to destroy their enemies, because it required them to do wrong; we reject a plan because it requires us to do right, and to destroy wrong.

Another such battle had captured his spirit early in his career. He had gone to Greece to fight for her liberty from the Ottoman Empire. He wrote home from Greece in 1826:

I came to Greece to serve her, and not to make money, and I shall stick by her to the last. The affairs of the country do not go on so well as could be wished. We could beat off the Turks, let them come on as thick as they pleased, but this season they have sent an army of disciplined Arabians from Egypt, before whom the Greeks cannot stand . . . They are now besieging Missolonghi, a very important town (fortified mostly by poor Lord Byron), and if they take it things will go badly.

But he stayed, because "I have received the appointment of physician and surgeon to the hospital at Napoli [Nauplion, Greece], where I have an excellent opportunity of perfecting myself in my profession. I am still a young man and a young doctor, and I look upon information as of more value than money."

After the Greek campaigns, he established himself in Boston, where the "perfection of his profession" meant his work with the blind. Nevertheless, four years later, he was back in Paris, to study the causes of optic degeneration. When the July Revolution of 1830 broke out, his friendship with the Marquis de Lafayette, its patriarchal leader, almost cost him his life. While in Germany, Howe fell afoul of the antirevolutionary Prussians, who placed him in solitary confinement for bringing French-American aid to Polish soldiers stranded in squalid refugee camps. Howe wrote to his Parisian colleagues from prison:

> I'll be cool then and let you know where and how I am—snug enough, between four granite walls, in a wee bit cell, fast barred and bolted, and writing by the light which comes in from a little grated window, or air-hole, eight feet from the floor. I am kept in perfect seclusion; not a newspaper is allowed . . . not a sound disturbs my meditations, save the sentinel's heels as he paces up and down the corridor.

He obtained some German works on the education of the blind—"I did not know of their existence in France," he wrote from prison. "I hope if pen and paper are granted me here to translate some good things. If by the next packet you hear not of my liberation, then do all that can be done for me." Fortunately, a Franco-American committee in Paris, which included the Marquis de Lafayette, James Fenimore Cooper, and Samuel F. B. Morse, prevailed on the State Department to mobilize the Prussians into releasing Howe. The doctor was transported to the nearest border in a sealed post wagon, accompanied by two policemen. Jolting over rough byroads, Howe "suffered the torments of the damned . . . until a copious vomiting relieved my pains. I could not persuade them to get me a glass of water. My strength of constitution however enabled me to undergo the journey, which lasted six days and during which I was subjected to a thousand vexations."

On his return to Paris, Lafayette wrote Howe: "I warmly feel it is the duty of the American Committee in Paris to offer you a vote of thanks for the manner in which our instructions have been understood and executed to the great comfort of the Polish soldiers, to the credit of the American name and to the gratification of every good Heart and sound Mind." A grateful Howe recalled that he was even more pleased by the cries of "Vive l'Amérique!" and "Vive la France!" that he heard from exiled Poles on his rattling journey over Prussian roads.

The Prussians had neither officially arrested Howe nor preferred charges; they offered no apologies. Many years later, however, when the King of Prussia gave him a gold medal "for philanthropic achievements in teaching the blind," Howe had the curiosity to weigh it and found that its value, in money, was equal to the sum which he had been forced to pay the Prussians for his prison board and lodging in 1832.

In Boston, Howe became perhaps the first American physician to interest himself in the study of what we would nowadays call "special education." The first school for the blind, the Perkins Institution, of Watertown, Massachusetts, was his creation, and Laura Bridgman (the Helen Keller of the abolitionists) was his student. But his work with the blind never preempted his more general social concerns. His commitment to the abolitionist movement culminated on September 5, 1861, when—in the words of the minutes—"A meeting called for this day was held at Dr. Howe's room, 20 Bromfield Street, to take into consideration measures tending to the Emancipation of the Slaves as a War Policy." Those attending included Wendell Phillips, James Freeman Clarke, William Lloyd Garrison—the usual cohort of Boston abolitionists.

Dr. Howe was not only active in support of emancipation and in the independence of Greeks, Poles, and Italians. After the Civil War, he also became committed to the cause of equal rights for women. In this movement, as in the cause of abolition, he found more than an equal partner. Julia Ward Howe, in a lifetime of meliorist zeal, had become a formidable force in the women's suffrage movement, a ubiquitous lecturer for progressive causes, and a perfectly sound, professional poet. It was in this role that she accompanied Dr. Holmes when he next visited New York to read appropriate verses at the seventieth birthday celebration of William Cullen Bryant in 1864. Bryant had been a founder of the campaign for Central Park in the 1840s; together with Washington Irving and other literati he had written that proposal for a "good healthy pair of lungs for the entire population." He was also a fellow abolitionist and, at the time, editor of the New York *Evening Post*. His calls in 1862 for a swift Union victory became almost as popular as "The Battle Hymn of the Republic."

> *Strike for that broad and goodly land!*
> *Blow after blow, till men shall see*
> *That Might and Right move hand in hand,*
> *And glorious must their triumph be!*

The audience that evening also heard Dr. Holmes. Among the celebrants were a good number of abolitionists and sanitarians who had heard Holmes before on the need for prevention of disease—rather than its treatment by harsh, useless remedies. He had assured those folks that, while medical science could take the huddled masses of new Americans under her wing, curative medicine was powerless against the epidemics of yellow fever, typhoid, dysentery, or cholera brought in by Irish and German immigrants. Science—in her female form—was gracious, but futile.

> *When in gracious hand are seen*
> *The dregs and scum of earth and seas,*
> *Her kindness counting all things clean*
> *That lend the sighing sufferer ease;*
>
> *Though on the field that Death has won,*
> *She saves some stragglers in retreat;—*

> *These single acts of mercy done*
> *Are but confessions of defeat.*

Those defeats could be avoided by strict attention to sanitarian principles: wide-open public spaces, clean water, proper sewage, a sanitation corps, and parks. Parks in the center of cities. Parks like the one on which doctor and poet, sculptor and reformer have left their mark: Dalton and Bryant, Stebbins and Saint-Gaudens, Olmsted and Vaux.

> *God lent his creatures light and air,*
> *And waters open to the skies;*
> *Man locks him in a stifling lair,*
> *And wonders why his brother dies!*

Central Park, that monument to abolition and sanitation, that clear space full of light and air, with waters open to the skies, is a reminder of what *can* be done for crowded cities. When the long fight of the sanitarians against slavery was over in the rural South, they turned their attention to preventing the newer epidemics of the North. They anticipated that the "dregs and scum of earth and seas"—those huddled masses yearning to breathe free—would eventually transform the center of American cities. They began to tackle the urban predicaments of a postwar era: teeming streets and squalid housing, malnutrition and infection. Instead of throwing up their hands at the problems of cities, or describing them as *cloacinas* (Jefferson's term for New York), they set about widening the streets, clearing the slums, and keeping the water clean. As a result, when the last pandemic of cholera swept westward through Europe in 1892, when the disease devastated Hamburg and Genoa—the ports from which immigrants sailed to America—only ten cases of cholera appeared in

New York, whose population had grown to 1.5 million. That epic of prevention began with the sanitarian vision of Central Park, an open space where the lawns were green, the bridges handsome, the water beautiful, and the swans forever elegant in their deportment.

8. COLONELS HIGGINSON AND SHAW IN SOUTH CAROLINA

HEADQUARTERS, ARMY OF THE POTOMAC September-ber 19 1862 *We have had a severe fight day before yesterday [Antietam]—a good many officers on our side wounded because the men in some brigades behaved badly. Frank Palfrey is wounded, not seriously,—Paul Revere, slightly wounded,—Wendell Holmes shot through the neck, a narrow escape, but not dangerous now—Hallowell badly hit in the arm, but he will save the limb—Dr. Revere is killed,—also poor Wilder Dwight. . . . Bob Shaw was struck in the neck by a spent ball, not hurt at all.*

> —Captain Charles Russell Lowell, 2nd Mass. Cavalry,
> letter to his mother

For some who fought it and for many who could not, the Civil War was always about slavery. After Fort Sumter, many in the North went willingly to war for Webster's "Union and Liberty, Now and Forever, One and Inseparable," while Southerners signed up by the brigade to defend Calhoun's "Liberty, Justice, and the Constitution." But even before Antietam, the battle that permitted Lincoln to proclaim Emancipation, at least three groups of Americans knew that slavery was the major issue of the war: Yankee abolitionists, Southern Cavaliers, and every black in America. Six years before Antietam, Emerson was already convinced. He wrote to Thomas Carlyle that "the fight of slave and freeman is drawing nearer, the question is sharply, whether slavery, or whether freedom shall be abolished."

105

Shortly after Antietam, Sarah Shaw, a fervid abolitionist and mother of Robert Gould Shaw, wrote to her son urging him to accept the colonelcy of the 54th (Free Black) Regiment of Massachusetts volunteers: "I feel as if God had called you up to a holy work . . . when the most important question is to be solved that has been asked since the world began. I know the task is arduous, but it is God's work." It was quite a maternal load to place on the shoulders of a twenty-five-year-old! But young Captain Shaw was already a veteran of Antietam, as his brother-in-law, Charles Russell Lowell, reported. It took Shaw a few days to decide, but after some vacillation he accepted his charge and by February 1863, Massachusetts was able to field a regiment of free black volunteers led by no fewer than a dozen Harvard officers.

It would seem a foregone conclusion that Robert Gould Shaw would accept the leadership of a black regiment. He was brought up in a household committed to social reform in pursuit of God's work on earth. His parents, Francis George and Sarah Shaw—heirs to great commercial wealth—had moved to West Roxbury in 1841 to attend classes at the Brook Farm commune. They also contributed a good portion of the family fortune to its founding. As Hawthorne described it in *The Blithedale Romance*, the Brook Farmers had joined for the purpose of "showing mankind the example of a life governed by other than the false and cruel principles, on which human society has all along been based . . . to offer up the earnest toil of our bodies, as a prayer, no less than an effort, for the advancement of our race." These notions were one expression of the Transcendental movement, which Colonel Lowell's uncle, James Russell Lowell, attributed to the Puritan spirit seeking a "new outlet and escape from forms and creeds which compressed rather than expressed it." The Transcendental Emerson was somewhat less sanguine about the dream of Brook Farm, calling it a "perpetual picnic," a "French Revolution in small, an Age of Reason in a patty-pan."

But slavery was no picnic-table subject for the Shaws and their fellow Brook Farmers. They were in dead earnest on the subject of abolition, so much so that a younger Robert Shaw had written to his mother in 1858, "Because I don't talk and think Slavery all the time, and because I get tired . . . of hearing nothing else, you say I don't feel with you, when I do." But despite young Shaw's lament, slavery was not the only concern of his family and friends. Sarah Shaw and her bosom companion the feminist Lydia Maria Child had sat with Margaret Fuller in the course of her "Conversations," *Kulturklätsche* for women that Fuller held to support herself after she quit teaching. Goethe and Fourier, idealism and reform were the topics of those splendid literary sessions, which attracted among others the wives of Emerson, Lowell, and Agassiz. For his part, Francis George Shaw had translated Pellarin's biography of Charles Fourier. Shaw *père* and *mère* were smitten in turn by Fourierist schemes of social planning and the Swedenborgian fervor of their fellow philanthropist Henry James the elder. Emerson again demurred, believing that Fourier and Swedenborg combined the worst aspects of mathematics and spiritualism, respectively. Fourierism may have come and gone, but abolition remained the Shaws' chief passion. With the Howes at Green Peace, they collected money and support for John Brown; with William Lloyd Garrison, they introduced Frederick Douglass to radical Boston society. Abolition and social experiment proved as irresistible as maternal pressure to a child of this circle.

Robert Gould Shaw's inevitable decision surprised no one. That February, Norwood Penrose (Pen) Hallowell, his arm healed after Antietam, wrote to his Harvard classmate and fellow battlefield veteran Oliver Wendell Holmes, Jr., "By a power as irresistible as fate I am drawn into the coloured regiment (54th) as Lt. Col. Would you take the majority, not that it would be offered you, but your name would command attention? Bob Shaw has accepted the colonelcy." Oedipally vexed with having his—and his father's—name command attention, Captain

Holmes declined, but one of Henry James's troubled younger sons, Garth Wilkinson James (Wilky) eagerly accepted a commission.

Wilky, who had been named after his father's English confidant, the Swedenborgian preacher John Garth Wilkinson, was little more than a hesitant schoolboy when he became adjutant of the 54th. It seems not unlikely that he went to war to avoid eclipse by his dazzling elder brothers, but his military career ended less than six months later. Wilky was badly wounded in the failed attack on Fort Wagner on July 18, 1863, in the course of which Robert Gould Shaw was killed and Pen Hallowell again wounded. Meanwhile, Wilky's brother William James sat out the war with an imaginary back injury, wondering what he would do with his life. A month after Fort Wagner, William wrote to a cousin: "I have four alternatives, Natural History, Medicine, Printing and Beggary." He inclined to natural history and Agassiz, with as little chance of beggary as of military service. Guilt reared its head as he watched Wilky brought back to Boston to lie in a stairwell in his father's house: "his wound is very large . . . he is the best abolitionist you ever saw, and makes a common one, as we are, feel very small and shabby."

By May 30, 1897, William James had already left his great mark on both medicine and printing, if not on natural history. By virtue of his eminence and that family connection with the 54th, James was asked by Colonel Henry Lee Higginson—who had by then married Ida Agassiz and become banker to all of Harvard—to speak at the dedication of the Robert Gould Shaw monument. The sculpture on Boston Commons by Augustus Saint-Gaudens presents Shaw and his men in defile, guided by an angel of God. It recalls that other memorable day in May when the 54th marched through Boston on its way to war. Young Colonel Shaw, the "blue-eyed child of fortune," in James's phrase, had ridden in the vanguard, the regiment, its band and colors cheered not only by his parents and their friends—

Frederick Douglass, the Howes, the Holmeses, the Garrisons and Carys—but also by a vast crowd of ordinary Bostonians gathered on the Commons. They had been greeted by the abolitionist Governor Andrews, who presented the regiment with their colors, and hoped that "we not only see the germs of the elevation of a downtrodden and despised race, but a great and glorious future . . . when right and justice shall govern our beloved country."

Among the troops was Corporal James Henry Gooding, a black volunteer. He was one of the literate free blacks who worked on whaling ships out of New Bedford; he had traveled around the world. He was also a fledgling poet and correspondent whose dispatches from the regiment were published in the New Bedford *Mercury*. He described the mood in the ranks of the 54th on May 18, 1863:

> There is not a man in the regiment who does not appreciate the difficulties, the dangers, and maybe ignoble death that awaits him if captured by the foe [the Confederacy refused to recognize blacks as soldiers and threatened to hang all captives], and they will die upon the field rather than be hanged like a dog; and when a thousand men are fighting for a very existence, who dare say them men won't fight determinedly? The greatest difficulty will be to stop them.

Among those who rode to see the 54th off on that fervid day in May were Colonel Shaw's handsome sister, Josephine, and her fiancé, Colonel Charles Russell Lowell, sparkling in the blue-and-gold uniform of the 2nd Massachusetts Cavalry. The young William James wrote to his cousin, "I looked back and saw their faces and figures against the evening sky and they looked so young and victorious, that I, much gnawed by questions as to my own duty of enlisting or not, shrank back—they had not seen me—from being recognized."

Years later, Robert Lowell, who had sat out the war against

Hitler, remembered William the philosopher, rather than Charles, his kinsman, when he brooded on the Saint-Gaudens monument in *For the Union Dead* (1964):

> *Two months after marching through Boston*
> *half the regiment was dead;*
> *at the dedication,*
> *William James could almost hear the bronze Negroes breathe.*

Well, not quite. On the day after the dedication ceremonies in 1897, William described them to his brother Henry: "The monument is really superb, certainly one of the finest things of this century. Read the darkey [Booker T.] Washington's speech, a model of elevation and brevity. The throng that struck me most in the day was the faces of the old 54th soldiers . . . The heavy animal look entirely absent, and in its place the wrinkled, patient, good old darkey soldiers." Henry James must have received the news with a sympathetic ear; over the years he had suffered from his own imaginary injury, an "obscure hurt," the Jamesian onset of which coincided with news of Fort Sumter. Always disturbed by the strange, Henry had glum forebodings as he watched the 54th training outside Boston in May 1863: "though our sympathies . . . were, in the current phrase, all enlisted on behalf of that race that had sat in bondage, it was impossible for the mustered presence of more specimens of it, and of *stranger* than I had ever seen together, not to make the young men who were about to lead them appear sacrificed" (italics added).

The sacrifice came on July 18, 1863. The 54th stormed Fort Wagner, one of the bastions that guarded Charleston Harbor. Corporal Gooding reported the news to his New Bedford readers:

> You may all know Fort Wagner is the Sebastopol of the re-
> bels; but we went at it, over the ditch and on to the parapet

through a deadly fire; but we could not get into the fort. We met the foe on the parapet with the bayonet—we were exposed to a murderous fire from the batteries of the fort, from our Monitors and our land batteries as they did not cease firing soon enough. Mortal men could not stand such a fire and the assault on Wagner was a failure. . . . At the first charge the 54th rushed to within twenty yards of the ditches, and, as might be expected of raw recruits, wavered—but at the second advance they gained the parapet. The color bearer of the State colors was killed on the parapet. Col Shaw seized the staff when the standard bearer fell, and in less than a minute after, the Colonel fell himself. When the men saw their gallant leader fall, they made a desperate effort to get him out, but they were either shot down, or reeled in the ditch below.

The next day, the ditch was filled with many of the 272 dead Union soldiers of the 600 who had made the charge. The Confederate officer commanding, General Johnson Hapgood, saw to it that Shaw's body was covered with twenty of his men. The general's remark, "Let him lie there with his niggers," has come down in legend as a fit epitaph for a son of the Boston Shaws.

When Fort Wagner was abandoned by the Confederates later that summer, it was proposed that Shaw's remains be exhumed and returned to Massachusetts. Francis George Shaw instructed the regimental surgeon, Dr. Lincoln Stone, to permit no such move: "We mourn over our loss and that of the regiment, but find nothing else to regret in Rob's life, death or burial. We would not have his body removed from where it lies surrounded by his brave and devoted soldiers if we could accomplish it by a word . . . his remains may *not* be disturbed." Gooding and the men of the 54th raised money for a monument, and some wanted it planted at the parapet where Shaw fell. Gooding disagreed and wrote back to New Bedford arguing the case for a monument to Shaw in Boston: "The first to say that a black was a man, let her [Massachusetts] have the first monument raised by black men's money, upon her old rocks." The community raised a thousand dollars, but a generation passed before the monument was built, and by then no one remembered the original donors.

Shaw has left another kind of monument: his volume of letters. They constitute a condensed *Bildungsroman* which tells how a blue-eyed child of fortune became a formidable leader of men in the course of six short months. One episode stands out. Two weeks before the attack on Fort Wagner, Shaw attended a July 4 celebration at St. Helena's Island, presided over by the Rev. Lynch, a black abolitionist minister from Baltimore. Shaw was accompanied by a perky black schoolmistress from Philadelphia, Charlotte Forten, and by Colonel Thomas Wentworth Higginson. All three left accounts of the event and all three jibe; Shaw's is perhaps the most affecting because we know what is coming. First on horseback, then dismounted, the three had watched the scene:

> Here were collected all the freed slaves on this island listening to the most ultra abolition speeches, that could be made, while two years ago, their masters were still here, the lords of the soil & of them. Now they all own a little themselves, go to school, to church, and work for wages. It is the most extraordinary change. Such things oblige a man to believe that God isn't far off.

✳

Shaw, Higginson, and Forten were in South Carolina as part of a wartime maneuver that began as a blockade and turned into a bold social experiment. Union troops had landed early in the war to occupy the strategic Sea Islands off South Carolina. Their landing was perhaps the first time in human history that soldiers had made landfall on a strange shore to liberate rather than enslave another race. One such landfall was made on the eastern shore of America early on the morning of November 24, 1862, and is described in Thomas Wentworth Higginson's classic *Army Life in a Black Regiment* (1870). Higginson, a cousin of Henry Lee Higginson, had been newly appointed as colonel of the 1st South Carolina Volunteers, the first unit of emancipated slaves to be armed by the Union:

> . . . no sail, until at last appeared one light-house, said to be Cape Romaine, and then a line of trees and two distant vessels and nothing more. The sun set, a great illuminated bubble, submerged in one vast bank of rosy suffusion; it grew dark; after tea all were on deck, the people sang hymns; then the moon set, a moon two days old, a curved pencil of light, reclining backwards on a radiant couch which seemed to rise from the waves to receive it. Towards morning the boat stopped, and when I came on deck, before six, Hilton Head lay on one side . . . stars were still overhead, gulls wheeled and shrieked, and the broad river rippled duskily towards Beaufort. Reporting to General Saxton, I had the luck to encounter a company of my destined command, marched in to be mustered into the United States service.

The troops of that command, the general who mustered them into service, and the colonel who was to lead them were joined in a novel enterprise. For on those Union-held islands that commanded the shipping lanes of the Confederate cotton trade, abolitionist theory was put to test by fire. The South Carolina islands were rich in plantations and awash in cotton; the Union decided not only to employ and to educate the slaves who had worked there, but also to arm them. Yankee officers like Rufus Saxton, Charles T. Trowbridge, Thomas Wentworth Higginson, Robert Gould Shaw, and Norwood Penrose Hallowell overcame the objections of Copperhead and skeptic to train the black regiments that eventually helped turn the tide of the Civil War. They also participated in a meliorist experiment that permitted educated black and white Americans to work together.

The Sea Islands of South Carolina were a new world not only for Higginson but for most of the Yankee Roundheads. The rich tropical scenery, the sloping beaches, the abandoned plantations, the exotic mix of freed slaves, the so-called contrabands of war, missionaries, storekeepers, and cotton traders moved the young Union officers to florid prose. Charles Francis Adams, Jr., wrote to his brother, Henry Adams, from Port Royal:

> Nothing can destroy the charm of the long plantation avenues with the heavy grey moss drooping from branches fresh with young leaves, while the natural hedges for miles along are fragrant with wild flowers. As I canter along these never end-ing avenues I hear sounds and see sights enough to set the ornithologist and sportsman crazy. The mocking bird is never silent, and the varieties of plumage are to the uninitiated in-finite, while hares and grey squirrels seem to start up under your horse's feet; wild pigeons and quail from every field, and duck and plover from every swamp . . .

The passage supports Edmund Wilson's contention that Henry Adams was a literary genius, but that Charles wrote bet-ter. The tropical shores contained not only hare and squirrel, duck and plover but also natives. The plantation owners having fled, the islands were populated by freed or escaped slaves who needed to be dealt with in humane fashion and whose fragile situation wanted relief. Adams, scion of presidents, had no great hopes for the Negro's ability to cope. He complained to Henry in England that the government had sent commercial agents to the islands and private philanthropies had sent missionaries. Ad-ams had little use for either group. The agents, he reported, made the freed slaves earn their bread by picking cotton for Union stores, while the missionaries taught them to read in re-turn for sermons. Adams predicted "divers results, among which are numerous jobs for agents and missionaries, small comfort to the negroes and heavy loss to the Government." Skeptical in the extreme as to the results of emancipation, Adams nevertheless affirmed:

> I am a thorough believer in this war. I believe it to have been necessary and just. I believe that from it will flow great blessings to America and to the Caucasian race. I believe the area of freedom will by it be immensely expanded in this country . . . but for the African I do not see the same bright future. He is the foot-ball of passion and accident, and the gift of freedom may prove his destruction. Still the experiment should and must be tried and the sooner it is tried the better.

The experiment eventually hinged on making soldiers out of the "Africans," and splendid soldiers many of them became. Higginson recounts how those former slaves were turned into an effective soldiery with pluck, good spirits, and a dash of bravery. He describes what happened after he got his regiment into fighting shape. They had been assigned the task of bottling up Confederate ships in the waterways of South Carolina and of launching expeditions to free yet more slaves who worked the plantations along its rivers. His account of an early morning landing is perhaps as meaningful as the news of an American army landing on Omaha Beach almost a century later. *Pace* revisionists, it is no accident that the name of Columbus is evoked:

> The only course was to land, under cover of the guns. As the firing ceased . . . I went ashore with a boat-load of troops at once. The landing was difficult and marshy. The astonished negroes tugged us up the bank and gazed on us as if we had been Cortez and Columbus. From emerald fields, they kept arriving by land much faster than we could come by water; every moment increased the crowd, the jostling, the mutual clinging on that miry foothold. Presently they began to come from their houses also, with their little bundles on their heads; then with larger bundles. Old women . . . would move on till

irresistibly compelled by thankfulness to dip down for another invocation.

Colonel Higginson wrote in the peroration of his book, "We who served with the black troops have this peculiar satisfaction, that whatever dignity or sacredness the memories of the war may have to others, they have more to us. . . . We had touched the pivot of the war. . . . Til the blacks were armed, there was no guaranty of their freedom. It was their demeanor under arms that shamed the nation into recognizing them as men." Higginson never forgot "that morning sunlight, those emerald fields, those thronging numbers." He remained convinced to the end of his days that the deed of "that day of jubilee was worth all it cost, and more." It was the faith of an abolitionist.

Cultural historians have traced the origins of the abolitionist movement in New England to several sources, but three stand out: Puritan faith, Transcendentalist hope, and Universalist charity. It is not surprising, therefore, to find that General Rufus Saxton, to whom T. W. Higginson reported in South Carolina, had in 1841 written for Margaret Fuller's *The Dial* an essay entitled "Prophecy—Transcendentalism—Progress." Prophecy was Saxton's reference to the Old Testament promise of a New Jerusalem in the New World. Transcendentalism stood for Emersonian idealism. Progress for Saxton meant Universalist equality, and that called for the abolition of slavery. The officers he recruited to work with black soldiers were abolitionists—if not Transcendentalists—to the core. His choice of Higginson was inevitable.

After Harvard, Thomas Wentworth Higginson was ordained as a Unitarian minister but even the gentle theology of that sect was too confining. He left Boston to found the Free Church in Worcester; its informal strictures later became models for the Universalist and Ethical Culture movements. In May 1854, Higginson, Dr. Howe, and others battered in the door of a Boston courthouse to rescue the fugitive slave Anthony Burns. Shortly thereafter Higginson went to Kansas and won his battle spurs at the side of John Brown. After military service and wartime wounds came his *Army Life in a Black Regiment* and an honorable career in American letters. Emancipation achieved, he worked the platforms with Samuel Gridley and Julia Ward Howe, with Lucy Stone and the Blackwells, to advocate votes for women and to preach Universalist tolerance and the concern of an Ethical Culture. It is therefore not surprising that Higginson wrote the first full-length biography of Margaret Fuller (1881), or that he became the first editor of Emily Dickinson's poems. Indeed, it was his "Letter to a Young Contributor" for *The Atlantic Monthly* that led Dickinson to send him a few of her poems, and to begin their correspondence of mutual trust. Higginson understood that this lonely spinster of Amherst entertained the "hope, always rather baffled, that I should afford some aid in solving her abstruse problem of life." In a very real sense, he fulfilled that hope by making her private poems public for all time.

Higginson, in his role as a regimental commander, moved with tact and understanding in the new multiracial society of the liberated Sea Islands. In her journal, Charlotte Forten, a young black abolitionist and schoolteacher, confirms Higginson's upbeat account of that first venture in racial equality. Her journal also records her chaste flutters with Robert Gould Shaw two weeks before Fort Wagner. "There is something girlish about him, and yet I never saw anyone more manly. To me he is a thoroughly lovable person. And there is something so exquisite about him. The perfect breeding, how evident it is. . . . We had a very pleasant talk on the moonlit piazza, and then went to the Praise house to hear the shout [gospel singing]." The next night he helped her on her horse, and after carefully arranging the folds of her riding skirt, told her that he would be pleased to receive her at his home. She rode off that night in the company of Pen Hallowell. After Fort Wagner, she set to work helping with the wounded of the 54th, both black and white,

and sighs to her diary how well Hallowell had looked that evening, and how badly wounded he was now. She learned from
Pen that Shaw had left her one of his horses "in case he fell."

Her account of a meeting with Colonel Higginson on New
Year's Day 1863 is the beginning of a set piece of Emancipation:

Thursday, January 1, 1863. The most glorious day this nation
has yet seen, *I* think. I rose early—an event here—and early
we started, with an old borrowed carriage and a remarkably
slow horse. Whither were we going? thou wilt ask. To the
ferry; thence to Camp Saxton, to the Celebration . . . Just as
my foot touched the plank, on landing, a hand grasped mine
and a well known voice spoke my name. It was my dear and
noble friend, Dr. Rogers [a Massachusetts army surgeon]. I
cannot tell you, dear diary, how delighted I was to see him;
how good it was to see the face of a friend from the North,
and such a friend. I think myself particularly blessed to have
him for a friend. Walking on a little distance I found myself
being presented to Col. Higginson, whereat I was so much
overwhelmed, that I had no reply to make to the very kind
and courteous little speech with which he met me.

The celebration at Camp Saxton was the announcement on
formerly Confederate soil of the Emancipation Proclamation. It
could not have happened but for Antietam, and certainly not
but for the party of abolition. It was prompted at least in part
by the sort of resolution passed in Dr. Howe's Boston cham-
bers: "to take into consideration measures tending to the Emancipation of the Slaves as a War Policy."

The proclamation was read to the black men of the 1st South
Carolina Volunteers. At about ten o'clock on New Year's Day
the people began to collect by land and over water in steamers
sent by General Saxton for the purpose; and from that time all
approaches were thronged. The ladies came on horseback and
in carriages, there were superintendents and teachers, officers,

and cavalrymen. The troops were marched to the neighborhood of the platform, and permitted to sit or stand, as at the Sunday services; the platform was occupied by ladies and various dignitaries; the band of the white 8th Maine played martial tunes. As Forten recounts, the words Higginson spoke at the celebration were "grand and glorious. He seemed inspired." As Higginson described it, the moment passes from history into literature:

Above, the great live-oak branches and their trailing moss; beyond the people, a glimpse of the blue river . . . Then the colors were presented to us by the Rev. Mr. French, a chaplain who brought them from the donors in New York. All this was according to the programme. Then followed an incident so simple, so touching, so utterly unexpected and startling, that I can scarcely believe it on recalling, though it gave the key-note to the whole day. The very moment the speaker had ceased, and just as I took and waved the flag, which now for the first time meant anything to these poor people, there suddenly arose, close beside the platform, a strong male voice (but rather cracked and elderly), into which two women's voices instantly blended, singing, as if by an impulse that could no more be repressed than the morning note of the song-sparrow:

> My Country, 'tis of thee,
> Sweet land of liberty,
> Of thee I sing!

People looked at each other, and then at us on the platform, to see whence came this interruption, not set down in the bills. Firmly and irrepressibly the quavering voices sang on, verse after verse; others of the colored people joined in; some whites on the platform began, but I motioned them to silence. I never saw anything so electric; it made all other words cheap; it seemed the choked voice of a race at last unloosed. Nothing could be more wonderfully unconscious; art could not have dreamed of a tribute to the day of jubilee that should be so affecting; history will not believe it; and when I came to speak of it, after it was ended, tears were everywhere . . . When they stopped, there was nothing to do for it but to speak, and I went on; but the life of the whole day was in those unknown people's song.

✹

Had abolitionists such as Francis and Sarah Shaw simply been urging their boys to wage God's war on earth, they would only have been preaching a Yankee-led jihad. Had they simply been appealing to altruistic motives, they would have enlisted only the sentimental. But since they tied the aims of Education and Enterprise to that of Emancipation, their cause in the eyes of the educated became that of the party of Puritan reason. Robert Gould Shaw hoped that former slaves would be free to "go to school, to church, and work for wages." School, church, and wages—and the first of these is school. The abolitionists won over many to their ranks by arguing that whereas slaves were condemned to remain dull, free men had the right to become educated and to think. It was a powerful argument. On August 10, 1862, a month before Antietam, Henry Lee Higginson of the Army of the Potomac wrote to his brother James, then studying in Germany: "We are fighting against slavery, present and future, and we are struggling for the right of mankind to be educated and to think: come and do your part." James came home, joined the Sanitary Commission, found it tame, and took up his sword with the 1st Massachusetts Cavalry.

Later that year, Emerson explained the entrepreneurial side of Emancipation to Thomas Carlyle. The proclamation, he was certain, would give the Union "free labor to fight with the Beast, and see if labor and barrels and baskets cannot find out that they pass more commodiously and surely to their port through free hands than through [unschooled] barbarians."

Despite their chivalric rhetoric, the economic aspects of ab-

olition were as clear to the Southern generals as to Ralph Waldo
Emerson. By considering slaves to be chattel, and by refusing
to grant them the rights either of soldiers or citizens, the South-
ern Cavaliers were fighting to preserve the feudal structure of
the Cotton Kingdom. That cultural divide remains with us:
Southern charm and Northern efficiency. But the treatment of
Shaw and his men, the threat of death to captured black soldiers
or to freed slaves—the contrabands of war who marched with
Union forces—showed the harsher face of Dixie charm. The
Southern generals knew that they were engaged in an economic
battle for the indentured labor of black men. Hood, Stuart, and
Lee knew as well as Emerson that the war was fought not only
over the issue of states' rights but also for "labor and bar-
rels and baskets." Were blacks to be considered men—as in
Massachusetts—they would merit wages. If blacks were property—as in Georgia—they *were* wages.

Two episodes illustrate the Southern terms of surrender for
blacks in time of war. On September 7, 1864, Major General
William Tecumseh Sherman, commander of the Union army
that had just occupied Atlanta, received a letter from his
opposite, General J. B. Hood, in reply to a proposal of a two-
day truce in the course of which the entire civilian population of central Atlanta would be expelled from the Union
perimeter. Sherman had explained to Hood that he wished
to contract his lines of defense, fortify the railhead, reduce
the need for occupation forces, and turn the city into a
"pure military garrison or depot." The civilians were to be ex-
ported south accompanied by household goods, baggage, and
servants "with the proviso that *no force shall be used towards
the blacks*" (italics added) to compel them to follow their masters. In a letter to Halleck, Chief of Staff in Washington, Sherman anticipated that these terms would be unpopular but
insisted that "war is war, and not popularity-seeking." Hood
reluctantly agreed to accept the evacuees but ended his letter
with an accusation:

And now, sir, permit me to say that the unprecedented measure you propose transcends, in studied and ingenious cruelty,
all acts ever before brought to my attention in the dark history of war. In the name of God and humanity, I protest,
believing that you will find that you are expelling from their
homes and firesides the wives and children of a brave people.

Sherman replied immediately:

You style the measures proposed "unprecedented," and appeal to the dark history of war for a parallel, as an act of
"studied and ingenious cruelty." . . . I say that it is kindness
to these families of Atlanta to remove them now, at once,
from scenes that women and children should not be exposed
to, and the "brave people" should scorn to commit their
wives and children to the rude barbarians who thus, as you
say, violate the laws of war, as illustrated in the pages of its
dark history. In the name of common-sense, I ask you not to
appeal to a just God in such a sacrilegious manner. . . . Talk
thus to the marines, but not to me, who have seen these
things, and who will this day make as much sacrifice for the
peace and honor of the South as the best-born Southerner
among you. If we must be enemies, let us be men, and fight
it out as we propose to do, and not deal in such hypocritical
appeals to God and humanity. God will judge us in due time.

Hood fired one last salvo. By its reference to race, this letter
gives the lie to those revisionists who deny today that the Civil
War was about slavery. "You say, 'let us fight it out like men.'
To this my reply is—for myself, and I believe for all the true
men, ay, and women and children, in my country—we will fight
you to the death! Better die a thousand deaths than submit to
live under you or your Government and *your negro allies!*" (italics added).

In the event, central Atlanta did become a Union garrison-
depot and Sherman marched to the sea. The phrase "Talk thus

to the marines" became "Tell it to the marines" as a taunting response to flummery, while war became—well—war; or hell, depending on which Sherman you read.

Sherman documents another Cavalier display by Hood. After the fall of Atlanta, and the Union army's drive to the sea, Hood retreated, but struck back at least once against an outnumbered detachment of Sherman's men. The following letters were exchanged:

HEADQUARTERS ARMY OF TENNESSEE IN THE FIELD, *October 12, 1864:* To the Officer commanding the United States Forces at Resaca, Georgia. SIR: I demand the immediate and unconditional surrender of the post and garrison under your command, and, should this be acceded to, *all white officers and soldiers* [italics added] will be paroled in a few days. If the place is carried by assault, no prisoners will be taken. Most respectfully, your obedient servant,

J. B. Hood, *General.*

To this, Colonel Weaver, then in command, replied:

HEADQUARTERS SECOND BRIGADE, THIRD DIVISION, FIFTEENTH CORPS, RESACA, GEORGIA, *October 12, 1864.* To General J. B. HOOD: Your communication of this date just received. In reply, I have to state that I am somewhat surprised at the concluding paragraph, to the effect that, if the place is carried by assault, no prisoners will be taken. In my opinion I can hold this post. If you want it, come and take it.

Sherman recalls that Hood, in fact, did not attempt an assault, but limited his attack to the above threat and moved on. The blacks, contrabands, freed slaves, drovers, and the rest moved on in the train of Sherman's advance. Sherman then swung seaward to South Carolina, the state that had started it all, to the

shores where freed slaves, black Yankees, and Boston Roundheads first fought the Cavaliers. And when Charleston finally
surrendered, Sherman's guns fired their great salutes over Fort
Sumter and over Fort Wagner, where Robert Gould Shaw remained buried in the ditch with his men of the 54th Massachusetts Volunteers. The days of the Cotton Kingdom were gone
with the wind.

9. COMMEMORATION AND WITCHCRAFT

On July 18, 1865, Harvard held a commemoration ceremony for those who had served and those who had died in the war. The list of speakers was both long and eminent. There were trumpets and processions, poems by Dr. Holmes and Mrs. Howe, prayers by Philip Brooks, and speeches in extenso from Governor Andrew, General Meade, and Ralph Waldo Emerson. The main event of the ceremonies, however, was a long ode in the classical style of Pindar by James Russell Lowell. As he confessed to Thomas Wentworth Higginson, it had been written in great haste and with wrenching toil; the ode scattered meter and line over a torrent of verse that ranged from paean to dirge. Nevertheless, it was a grand success at the time and has retained a place in American poetic literature. Lowell had warmed up for the task in an elegy for Robert Gould Shaw, remembering not only the colonel of the 54th but also his own kinsmen, Charles Russell Lowell and James Jackson Lowell: "I write of one, / While with dim eyes I think of three; / Who weeps not others fair and brave as he?"

In the "Commemoration Ode," he remembered the young Brahmins in a less personal vein:

> I sweep them for a paean, but they wane
>   Again and yet again
> Into a dirge, and die away, in pain.
>   In these brave ranks I only see the gaps,

125

Thinking of dear ones whom the dumb turf wraps,
Dark to the triumph which they died to gain . . .

It was a moving occasion for all. Victory had been won, but
at great cost, while the assassination of Lincoln, "our Martyr-
chief," in April hung over the nation and the ode. Yet, although
tinged with tragedy, it was a moment of high triumph, a moment
when "a rescued Nation sets / Her heel on treason and the
trumpet hears / Shout victory . . ." High triumph and national
tragedy were celebrated by high verse in classic meter.

Tragic moments tend to dissipate with time. Karl Marx had
written an essay for a progressive American weekly, *The Revolution*, entitled "The Eighteenth Brumaire of Louis Napoleon."
Its opening lines remain a fit verdict for the Second Empire and
have attained a life of their own: "Hegel remarks somewhere
that all facts and personages of great importance in world history occur, as it were, twice. He forgot to add: the first time as
tragedy, the second as farce." Hegel's remark is apposite to the
uses of commemoration in New England.

Tragedy was replayed as farce twenty-five years later, in the
course of another ceremony that honored the Harvard dead.
Major Henry Lee Higginson had given a drained flatland across
the Charles River to the university. His proviso was that the
grounds were to be used as a playing field dedicated to six
friends who numbered among the Union dead: Dr. Edward
Barry Dalton, Charles Russell Lowell, James Jackson Lowell,
James Savage, Stephen George Perkins, and Robert Gould Shaw.
In his speech at the dedication in 1890, Higginson first rehearsed
the biographies of the dead Harvard men; he then addressed the
living with advice on how to behave on the football field:

But, in your games there is just one thing you cannot do,
even to win success. You cannot do one tricky or shabby
thing. Translate tricky and shabby—dishonest and ungentle-
manly. Princeton is not wicked, Yale is not base . . . Mates,

the Princeton and the Yale fellows are our brothers. Let us beat them fairly if we can, and believe that they will play the game just as we do.

The game that Higginson had played to a successful conclusion was the industrial expansion of America. The twenty-five years that elapsed between the two Harvard commemorations witnessed an unprecedented spurt of industrial and territorial development in the United States. Having done good, many of the Brahmins began to do very well indeed. Whereas antebellum fortunes had been founded on shipping and trade, the post-Civil War boom was founded on rails, raw materials, and finance. Charles Francis Adams became a railway and financial tycoon; he ended up chairman of the Union Pacific and treasurer of Harvard. As might be expected in Boston, such commercial success followed closely one's family ties. About the time Major Higginson married Ida Agassiz, John Quincy Shaw, uncle of Robert Gould Shaw, married her sister Pauline Agassiz. Major Higginson's brother-in-law, Alexander Agassiz, and Quincy Shaw struck it rich "beyond the wildest dreams of copper men" in the Calumet and Hecla mines of Michigan. News of the mines spread, and soon all the first families in Boston made secondary fortunes in copper shares. Based on this success, Higginson and his brother James founded the investment banking firm of Lee, Higginson. They went on to manage the finances of every Brahmin family in the book and of the Harvard endowment. The Ward branch of the abolitionist Howes became Baring's bank in New York. Even the two youngest James brothers, Wilky and Rob, wet their entrepreneurial feet in a profitless Florida cotton plantation.

Before the war, Emerson had been as much an enthusiast of trade as of the submarine cable. He contended that trade was the principle of liberty; that it had settled America and destroyed feudalism. He predicted that it would abolish slavery. In the Reconstruction era, Emerson got what he asked for. All those telegraph cables were made of copper; the metal was mined in the West and the proceeds flowed eastward. East and West, trade was in the saddle, reform was left to women and the intelligentsia went to Europe. The sequel to Van Wyck Brooks's *The Flowering of New England* is appropriately titled *New England: Indian Summer.*

Things went not much better in science or medicine. In 1870, Dr. Holmes's clinical colleague James Clark White urged that rigorous standards of laboratory and bedside teaching—matching those of Paris, Berlin, or Vienna—be introduced at the Harvard Medical School. He viewed the departure of American students for medical schools of the Continent as a reproach to America:

> When I find the young men of Europe flocking to our shores and crowding our native students from their seats and from the bedside, when the fees of our best lecturers are mostly paid in foreign coin, and when thousands of wealthy invalids from across the sea fill the waiting-rooms of our physicians, then I will confess that I am wrong, and that of the two systems of education ours is the best. Until then I shall seek in the spirit and working of their schools the secret of their success, the cause of our failings.

His plea went unanswered. Not until Johns Hopkins put together a university, a hospital, *and* a medical school in 1893 was there an institution standing on these shores that matched the best of Europe. While the bacteriological revolution was under way in Europe, no medical discovery of major import came from the New World. Nothing matched those three great antebellum discoveries of anesthesia (1846, Morton), the cause of puerperal sepsis (1842, Holmes), and the mechanism of gastric digestion (1832, Beaumont).

The attenuation of intellectual vigor after the war was accompanied by a loss of belief in the power of human reason, a failure of nerve after a heroic age. If New England had flowered in the first half of the century, it was because the rational, skeptical outlook of Holmes, Lowell, and Emerson had expanded the narrow ordinates of Puritanism. Mild Concord or subtle Cambridge replaced harsh Salem at the center of the Yankee conscience, but that literary flowering came to an end at Appomattox. In this sense, Lowell's "Commemoration Ode" may be read as an elegy not only for the Union dead but also for the American Renaissance.

Of that proud company of meliorists, Unitarians, and abolitionists who had made Boston the temporary Athens of America, Lowell was perhaps the most cosmopolitan. He succeeded Longfellow as professor of modern languages at Harvard; he was the first editor of *The Atlantic Monthly* and *The North American Review*; he later became American minister to Spain and to the Court of St. James's. The poetry and criticism he wrote were good enough for contemporaries to rank him with Emerson, Longfellow, Whittier, Holmes, and Hawthorne among the lions of the Saturday Club. In our century his seat at the table of American letters has been occupied successively by Edmund Wilson and Gore Vidal; Lowell's writings might be said to fuse the authority of the former with the wit of the latter, informed by a generosity to his fellow Americans that may have eluded his successors.

Lowell's generation had watched the blood of its sons shed for the cause of reason and Emancipation at Cedar Mountain, Antietam, and Fort Wagner. In the words of Oliver Wendell Holmes, Jr., the young Roundheads had been "touched with fire." Having defeated slavery at such cost, the Brahmins of Lowell's generation were unwilling to let dumb credulity disturb the steady flow of social progress. Lowell's "Commemoration Ode" may therefore also be read as a plea for a postwar America ruled by a new kind of active reason. It evoked Pindar to praise "truth in action," a Harvard version of deed not creed:

To-day our Reverend Mother welcomes back
*   Her wisest Scholars, those who understood*
The deepest teaching of her mystic tome,
*   And offered their fresh lives to make it good:*
*   No lore of Greece or Rome*
No science peddling with the names of things,
Or reading stars to find inglorious fates,
*   Can lift our life with wings . . .*
*   But rather far that stern device,*
The sponsors chose that round thy cradle stood
*   In the dim, unventured wood,*
*   The VERITAS that lurks beneath*
*   The letters' unprolific sheath. . . .*

Lowell was confident that VERITAS would be reborn in the Reconstruction era; that study of the arts would no longer be confined to the lore of Greece and Rome, that science would do better than peddle the names of things. His tribute to the Harvard dead continued the theme:

Many loved Truth and lavished life's best oil
*   Amidst the dust of books to find her . . .*
Virtue treads paths that end not in the grave;
No ban of endless night exiles the brave.

But it was his epitaph for Lincoln, three months dead, that put his ode into the anthologies: "Sagacious, patient, dreading praise, not blame / New birth of our new soil, the first American." With Lincoln enshrined, abolition a fact, the Union preserved, Lowell was encouraged that a stiff dose of VERITAS would overcome vulgar credulity. Its two aspects, fancy and terror, would vanish from among the educated classes as reason was joined to reform. He announced—prematurely, it turns out—that "such superstition as comes to the surface nowadays is the harmless [enthusiasm] of sentiment, pleasing itself with a fiction all the more because there is no more exacting reality behind it to impose a duty or demand a sacrifice."

(Jumping ahead quite a bit, we might note that his critique of the sentimental was endorsed—consciously or not—by Lionel Trilling one hundred years later in *Sincerity and Authenticity*. Commenting on the curious notion of R. D. Laing, Michel Foucault, et al. "that madness is health, that madness is liberation and authenticity," he pointed out that those who believe in authenticity "don't have it in mind to go mad, let alone insane —it is characteristic of the intellectual life of our culture that it fosters a form of assent which does not involve actual credence.")

In his ode, Lowell joined assent to credence, rhetoric to belief, in the service of reform and reason. But if reform faltered in the course of Reconstruction, reason fared well in academe. After the Civil War his university became an intellectual citadel that rivaled the academies of Greece and Rome; the anthem "Fair Harvard" confirmed the meliorist charge

> *Let not moss-cover'd error move thee by its side,*
> *While the world on truth's current glides by,*
> *Be the herald of light, and the bearer of love*
> *Till the stock of the Puritans die.*

Lowell and his fellow meliorists, heralds of light and the bearers of love, were certain that their countrymen would avoid the moss-covered errors of superstition. Truth would flow unimpeded until the stock of the Puritans died—or at least until one of that stock believed it worthwhile to tell the young heralds that "Princeton is not wicked, Yale is not base!"

❋

Three years after his "Commemoration Ode," Lowell struck again. In a major analysis of the Salem witch trials, he warned New England against the twin errors of sect and superstition.

Lowell defined one respect in which the Salem trials differed from all their predecessors. He pointed out that although some of the accused had been terrified into confessing, yet not one persevered in it but all died protesting their innocence, though an acknowledgment of guilt would have saved the lives of all. The accused also were not, as was commonly the case, abandoned by their friends. "In all the trials of this kind," he wrote, "there is nothing so pathetic as the picture of Jonathan Cary holding up the weary arms of his wife during her trial, and wiping away the sweat from her brow and the tears from her face."

Thirty women of Salem had been convicted of witchcraft and twenty put to death in an episode connected in some fashion to intense village factionalism. Young Ann Putnam, the poor slave girl Tituba, and a score of other defendants in the witchcraft trials confessed to out-of-body experiences, the sightings of great balls of fire, visions of multitudes in white glittering robes, and the sensation of flying out of body. Their reports mirrored those of the credulous in Lowell's postwar Boston, abuzz with "rappings, trance mediums, the visions of hands without bodies, the sounding of musical instruments without visible fingers, the miraculous inscriptions on the naked flesh, the enlivenment of furniture."

Those out-of-body experiences resemble those advocated by "alternative" healers of today, who describe wellness, as Jonathan Kabat-Zinn has, as "riding the waves, much as if I were lying on a rubber raft on the ocean and the waves were picking me up and taking me down . . . Lifting and falling away. Lifting and falling away." The Salem of Ann Putnam, the séance parlors of Beacon Hill, and today's yuppie ashrams share a common belief: accused and accuser, seer and seen, healer and healed are convinced that magic rules the body. Generally there is money to be made from that conviction.

The Salem witchcraft trials have been revisited recently, thanks to the speculation of Mary Kilbourne Matossian that many of the accused were not in league with the devil at all, but poisoned by ergot. Matossian has presented evidence that rye, infected by the fungus *Claviceps purpurea*, was the source of LSD-like hallucinogens and that lysergic acid or a related alkaloid brought out tics, paresthesias, and fanciful visions in the good citizens of Salem. But Salem's Rev. Parris held Satan and his coven responsible and, in consequence, hundreds were accused, nineteen of the alleged witches were hanged, and one unfortunate was pressed to death beneath a weight of stones for failure to plead.

The evidence for ergotism rests on several, albeit indirect and therefore not entirely compelling, lines of evidence: on a close concordance between the clinical syndrome of ergotism and the signs and symptoms of bewitchment in Salem; on cartographic evidence that all twenty-two of the afflicted households lay in moist hollows suitable for the cultivation of rye; on climatologic and botanical evidence for the likelihood that the rye of that year was contaminated by *Claviceps*; and on historical accounts of bread and grain discolored by the telltale carmine stain of *Claviceps*. But perhaps the most telling argument against chalking up "bewitchment" to a kind of mass hysteria and not to satanic compact is that small infants and cattle of the afflicted households also suffered and died of "fitts" and "unnatural causes."

Whether the seizures were caused by ergot or by Calvin, whether the visions were earth-borne or heaven-sent, the Salem witchcraft trials permitted Lowell to derive a lesson for 1868:

Credulity, as a mental and moral phenomenon, manifests itself in widely different ways, according as it chances to be the daughter of fancy or terror. The one lies warm about the heart as Folk-lore, fills moonlit dells with dancing fairies, sets out a meal for the Brownie . . . and makes friends with unseen powers as Good Folks; the other is a bird of night, whose shadow sends a chill among the roots of the hair: it sucks with the vampire, gorges with the ghoul and commits un-

cleanliness with the embodied Principle of Evil, giving up the
fair realm of innocent belief to a murky throng from the slums
and stews of the debauched brain.

Lowell's disdain for the zealots among his Puritan ancestors
was matched by his response to the authenticity babble of his
own time: "I look upon a great deal of the modern sentimen-
talism about Nature as a mark of disease," he wrote apropos
Thoreau. "It is a very shallow view that affirms trees and rocks
to be healthy and cannot see that men and their communities
are just as true to the laws of their organization and destiny."
In lines that might apply to his own descendant, Robert Lowell,
he scolded the hermit of Walden Pond for sitting out the Civil
War: "While he studied with respectful attention the minks and
woodchucks, his neighbors, he looked with utter contempt
on the august drama of destiny of which his country was
the scene." Lowell mocked Thoreau's claim of self-sufficiency,
knowing full well that the Thoreau family business was a prof-
itable pencil factory: "He [Thoreau] squatted on another man's
land; he borrows an ax; his boards, his nails, his bricks, his mortar, his books, his lamp, his fish-hooks, his plough, his hoe, all
turn state's evidence against him as an accomplice in the sin of
that artificial civilization which rendered it possible that such a
person as Henry D. Thoreau should exist at all."
    With Girondist impartiality, Lowell mistrusted the sectarians
of the right as much as the authentics of the left. His analysis
of the Salem witchcraft trials was based on economic principles.
Lowell traced Salem's obsession with witches to its roots in
Cromwellian doctrine and argued that witchcraft trials in England were an aspect of Calvinist belief. The trials were also
grounded in a tradition of contractual agreements among the
mercantile class. Lowell suggested that Christianity had invented
the soul as an individual entity to be "saved" or "lost"—like
money—and that the grosser wits of commerce came to treat
the soul as a "piece of property that could be transferred by

deed of gift or sale, duly signed, sealed and witnessed." He argued that the Salem model of witchcraft was based on an unholy contract between an individual witch and the Evil One. The success of their joint venture was to be judged by the number of souls they had pocketed: the ultimate bottom line, we might say. The trade that was in the saddle in Salem was the traffic in souls.

Dr. Holmes, like Lowell, was descended from Yankee preachers and had anticipated Lowell by tracing the Puritan obsession with saving souls to its commercial roots. In his 1853 centennial essay on Jonathan Edwards, Holmes took Edwards to task for his relentless insistence on the original sin of children. Edwards had preached in 1740: "As innocent as children seem to be to us . . . they are not so in God's sight, but are young vipers, and are infinitely more hateful than vipers, and are in a most miserable condition." Holmes analyzed this Puritan view of original sin in simple economic terms: Jonathan Edwards, Cotton Mather, and the rest of the Roundhead company believed that God (as Sovereign) had made a covenant (a contract) with Adam (as trustee) for the souls (the capital) of humankind. Holmes explained this in terms any Boston merchant could understand: "Every infant of the human race is entitled to one undivided share of the guilt and consequent responsibility of the Trustee to whom the Sovereign had committed its future and who invested it in a fraudulent concern."

While Holmes admired Edwards for his intellectual vigor, he scoffed at his literal reading of scripture: "The fruit, to taste which conferred an education, the talking ophidian, the many-centuried patriarch, the floating menagerie with the fauna of the drowning earth represented on its decks, the modelling of the first woman about a bone of the first man—all these things were to him . . . as real historical facts as the building of the pyramids." Holmes's descriptions of recurrent cycles in the religious revivals of Jonathan Edwards's Massachusetts remind one of the commodity futures market—or of ergotism. There are pages in

Edwards which sounded to Holmes like the accounts of an epidemic: faintings, convulsions, utter prostration, trances, visions
like those of delirium tremens—all those tantrums in search of
a devil. Holmes, whose tolerant, rational beliefs differed very
little from his friend Lowell's, concluded that it is less violence
to deify protoplasm than to diabolize the deity. Their alliance
evoked Lowell's tribute to Holmes:

> Master alike in speech and song
> Of fame's great antiseptic—Style,
> You with the classic few belong
> Who tempered wisdom with a smile.

No one could say that the wisdom of Jonathan Edwards was
tempered with a smile. But since wit is the guarantor of reason,
Lowell might have had Edwards in mind when he wrote, "Thoreau had no humor, and this implies that he was a sorry logi-
cian." Nor could one say that the wisdom of Thoreau was
tempered with a smile.

※

Lowell had it right: the enemies of sweet reason tend to be
humorless and saturnine. Mesmer was a gloomy man and Swedenborg was clinically depressed. Swedenborg saw the light—
literally—at the age of fifty-nine and found wisdom after an
episode of "vastation," the nineteenth-century euphemism for
adult depression. Emerson wrote of Swedenborg's metallurgic
epiphany: "He was let down through a column that seemed of
brass . . . that he might descend safely among the unhappy, and
witness the vastation of souls." Henry James, Sr., America's
most avid apostle of Swedenborg, also experienced an episode
of vastation and worked out its mysteries in a prolix treatise,
The Secret of Swedenborg (1859). Asked his opinion of James's
book, William Dean Howells replied, "He kept it." Years later
Justice Oliver Wendell Holmes, Jr., was not so terse. He wrote

to Sir Frederick Pollock that the elder James "was bothered with the thought that there were such things as science and rational sequence, and being altogether a man of dramatic *aperçus*, wasted pages trying to be what he wasn't meant for."

In 1863, James followed up his not so open *Secret* with another massive tract. Written while son Wilky was wounded at Fort Wagner and Robert Gould Shaw buried forever in its ditch, the book remained oblivious to the Civil War. It dealt instead with simpler issues such as the mutual influences of the heavens, the earth, and all living creatures and was therefore given the modest title of *Substance and Shadow; or Morality and Religion in Their Relation to Life: An Essay on the Physics of Creation.* Its morality owed much to Swedenborg and its physics was all Mesmer. As a comment on his father's work, the twenty-one-year-old William James designed a woodcut for the title page; it showed a man beating a dead horse. It was the last note of conscious humor sounded by any James but Alice.

Swedenborg may have been a dead horse then and he is a dead horse now, but Mesmer and his speckled band have remained remarkably alive. As we've learned from Robert Darnton's *Mesmerism and the End of the Enlightenment in France* (1968), there was a disturbing connection between the rise of Mesmeric belief and the end of the Enlightenment in both Europe and America. On both sides of the water, hard science and sharp thought provoked a backlash of soft science and dull thought. The result was a brew of Mesmeric fluid and Swedenborgian mind as the language of real science was appropriated by the mock. Both Mesmer, who began as a Viennese physician, and Swedenborg, who began as a Swedish metallurgist, slipped easily into the language of eighteenth-century physics; their tomes are filled with universal fluids and fields, forces of repulsion and attraction, terrestrial and animal magnetism. George Bush, no discernible relation of our recent leader, but a very discernible colleague of the elder James, published in 1847 a book entitled *Mesmer and Swedenborg.* He spelled out for

Americans the connection between the Barnum of animal magnetism and the Bailey of cosmologic love. For Bush as for James,
the relationship between flesh and spirit was elementary; it was,
so to speak, written in the stars. And the stars, then as now,
permitted one to deal with the dark side of the soul, with the
lonely self, with existential angst and with vastation. "His work
gives one the feeling of a sky full of stars," said Lowell of Thoreau, "astrology as yet, and not astronomy."

Alas, there are today many more astrologers than astrono-
mers in the United States. Americans still can't tell whether it's
the real turtle soup or only the mock. Our proliferation of crystal healers, visualizers, spiritual guides, homeopaths, gurus,
Ayurvedic practitioners, and herbalists is unmatched since the
era of Mesmer. Mesmer, of course, was only the most fashionable and successful practitioner among that squad of Svengalis
that serviced eighteenth-century salons. Darnton quotes a report
on the prevalence of false prophets in prerevolutionary France:
"Never, certainly, were Rosicrucians, alchemists, prophets, and
everything related to them so numerous and so influential. Conversation turns almost entirely upon these matters; they fill
everyone's thoughts; they strike everyone's imagination . . .
Looking around us, we see only sorcerers, initiates, necromancers, and prophets. Everyone has his own, on whom he counts."

Mesmer preached that all disease resulted from various obstacles to the flow of a magnetic fluid or energetic force in the
body. These obstacles could be overcome by massage or by
prodding certain vital "poles" of the body: a body scan, so to
speak. Mesmerists believed that when a "crisis" or "resistance"
was induced, the symptoms would dissipate and the "harmony"
of man with nature could be restored. The key to it all was an
energetic fluid that united everything. Darnton explains:

> Sitting around the tubs in circles, the patients communicated
> the fluid to one another by means of a rope looped about
> them all by linking thumbs and index fingers in order to form

a mesmeric "chain," something like an electric circuit . . . Soft music, played on wind instruments, a pianoforte, or the glass "harmonica" that Mesmer helped to introduce in France sent reinforced waves of fluid deep into [the patient's] soul. Every so often fellow patients collapsed, writhing on the floor, and were carried by Antoine, the mesmerist-valet, into the crisis room; and if his spine still failed to tingle, his hands to tremble, his hypochondria to quiver, Mesmer himself would approach, dressed in a lilac taffeta robe, and drill fluid into the patient from his hands, his imperial eye, and his mesmerized wand.

This report does not differ from the account Elizabeth Blackwell gave us over a generation later, nor, for that matter, of Mesmeric sessions held a generation after that one. We might say that constancy to this degree separates a cult or religion from Western science, which changes so rapidly that it often forgets its place on the page.

✳

It is in keeping with family tradition that William James toyed with the mechanics of Swedenborgian automatism and somnambulism in his psychological laboratory. James, a student of Dr. Holmes and a close friend of his son, became obsessed by the rational explanation of spiritual experience. On the occasion of James's death, and years after their paths had parted, Holmes the younger explained to Pollock why he had lost touch with his friend: "distance and other circumstance and latterly my little sympathy with his demi-spiritualism and pragmatism were sufficient cause. His reason made him skeptical and his wishes led him to turn down the light so as to give miracle a chance." Holmes, Jr., believed that James's anticipation of the "interstitial miracle" was only to be expected of one who had not bitten the bullet of secular reason.

William James's fascination with the occult led him to séances held by a Boston medium named Mrs. William J. Piper. He wrote to his sister Alice in England asking for a lock of her hair so that he might use it to conduct help from the spirit world. Sure enough, the hair was sent and advice was obtained. William James was convinced that he had tested the "conductive" power of material objects and confirmed the Swedenborgian correspondence of spirit and matter. Shortly thereafter, Alice confessed that the hair she had sent was not her own but that of her nurse, dead four years ago. "I thought it a better test of whether the medium is simply a mind reader or not." She had a less sanguine view of the spirit world than her brother, calling Mrs. Piper and her ilk "the curious spongy minds that sop it all up and lose all sense of taste and humour!"

Unfazed by the episode, William James became a president of the Society for Psychical Research. In *The Will to Believe* (1891), he used all the powers of his plangent rhetoric to defend its activities by pointing out the endurance of the clairvoyant tradition over the ages, "which lay broadcast over the surface of history. No matter where you open its pages, you find things recorded under the name of divinations, inspirations, demonical possessions, apparitions, trances, ecstasies, miraculous healings and productions of disease, and occult powers possessed by peculiar individuals." He remained on the lookout for that ecstasy in the cupboard and worried over the reductionism creeping in from Europe. He warned the theologians of Princeton against positivists "who keep chiming to us that amid the wreck of every other god and idol, one divinity still stands upright—that his name is Scientific Truth. But they are deluded." He rejected "the scientific conception of the world as an army of molecules" in favor of interstitial miracles to come.

A local periodical in Boston chided the Society for Psychical Research for its Mesmeric claims of clairvoyance through the universal ether. It complained that "soft-headedness and idiotic credulity are the band of sympathy in this society, and a general wonder sickness its dynamic principle." James answered by evoking the bona fides of those who had presided over it, including Drs. J. P. Langley of the Smithsonian Institution, Dr. Charles Richet of Charcot's *équipe*, and Sir William Crookes of the X-ray tube. We could augment his list with more recent rank-and-filers of spiritualism such as radium-sick Pierre Curie, Arthur Conan Doyle, William Butler Yeats, Ezra Pound, and much of the leadership of the National Socialist Party of Germany.

William James, the finest writer ever to have come out of the Harvard Medical School, believed at the end of his century what the New Age healers believe at the end of our own: that the "thunderbolt has fallen and that the orthodox belief in reductionist science has not only had its presumptions weakened, but the truth itself . . . decisively overthrown." Well, not really. Reductionist science in James's own field of medicine and physiology has had a decent run since its "overthrow" by Mrs. Piper. The sanitary revolution was followed by the bacteriological revolution, and this in turn was succeeded by the biological revolution, which I have called the Flowering of DNA. The results are easy to quantify: In 1920, at the end of the bacteriological revolution—and before the discovery of antibiotics—the average life expectancy in the United States was 53.6 years for males and 54.6 for females. By 1990, the life expectancy of males had increased to 71.8 and females to 78.8. There is no evidence that between 1920 and 1990 intervention from the spirit world had increased, nor—James and the spiritualists to the contrary—that the "truth itself" has been decisively overthrown.

The meliorist notion that sweet reason rather than dumb belief can change life for the better has already outlived both the tragedy of witchcraft and the farce of animal magnetism. Winthrop's city on the hill managed to survive the Salem witchcraft trials and the War of the Secession to become the Athens of America. Nor was the Flowering of New England forever choked by the weeds of Mesmer and Swedenborg. But unreason persists: the great war of our own mid-century has also been followed by a failure of nerve. The fans of witchcraft and aromatherapy are the distant heirs of the Salem elders, of Anton Mesmer and Jamesian clairvoyance. They are, after all, only throwbacks to Mrs. Piper and the Boston spiritualists, "curious spongy minds that sop it all up and lose all sense of taste and humour!"

Those fashionable folk who gave you Mesmer also gave you the original 18th of Brumaire: a takeover by a short despot in love with the military. Barras, displaced on that date by Napoleon, asked, "When this moment arrives, and the secretly conducted workings of opinion have reached their terms, where are the human resources which will be able to oppose it?" The answer was given by Dr. Holmes, whom Judge Pollock properly called "a right good optimist." Holmes gave a meliorist response to the Mesmeric medical practices of his day in his pamphlet *Homeopathy and Its Kindred Delusions*:

> As one humble member of [the medical] profession, which for more than two thousand years has devoted itself to the pursuit of the best earthly interests of mankind, always assailed and insulted from without by such as are ignorant of its infinite complexities and labors, always striving in unequal contest with [disease] not merely for itself but for the race and the future, I have lifted my voice against this lifeless delusion, rolling its shapeless bulk into the path of a noble science it is too weak to strike, or to injure.

10. SPINAL IRRITATION AND
THE FAILURE OF NERVE

In November 1864, the autumn between Gettysburg and Appomattox, Dr. Oliver Wendell Holmes, Parkman Professor of Anatomy and Physiology at the Harvard Medical School, traveled to New York by train. He was accompanied on his journey from Boston by Julia Ward Howe, then at the peak of her fame for "The Battle Hymn of the Republic." Mrs. Howe recalls that they did not stop talking for the entire journey and that never had she been more vastly entertained. Holmes and she were coming to the Century Association in order to read appropriate verses at the seventieth birthday celebration of William Cullen Bryant. All three, Holmes, Howe, and Bryant, were of broad sanguine temperament and good humor; they were also old friends. Bryant was not only an abolitionist and an enthusiast of Central Park but also a celebrated man of letters who edited the New York *Evening Post*. In addition, he was the lay leader of the Homeopathic Society.

Holmes was remarkably cordial that evening at the Century and recited his usual quota of amusing and completely forgettable quatrains. The next day's accounts of the occasion do not mention whether Bryant remembered that Dr. Holmes was the leading opponent of homeopathic practice in the United States. In Holmes's pamphlet *Homeopathy and Its Kindred Delusions* (1842) he had referred to Bryant's homeopathy as "a mingled mass of perverse ingenuity, of tinsel erudition, imbecile credulity, and of artful misrepresentation." But the evening went well,

143

presumably because a good dinner and a goodlier number of drinks can cause the lion to lie down with the lamb, even if the lamb won't get a good night's sleep.

Holmes had become Bryant's equal in literary renown by 1864; for almost a decade he had been featured in *The Atlantic Monthly*, America's most prestigious journal of arts and letters, where he had ample opportunity to temper his wisdom with a smile. He used almost every genre of humor to fill his monthly pieces, resorting often to the lowliest of them all, the pun. Holmes had himself complained in *The Autocrat* that "people who make puns are like wanton boys that put coppers on the railroad tracks. They amuse themselves and other children, but their little trick may upset a freight train of conversation for the sake of a battered witticism." (Unfortunately for the sage of Boston, his own puns seem battered indeed. He had few regrets that his ancient family home in Cambridge was to be razed to provide new buildings for Harvard. He called it a case of "justified domicide." He saluted John L. McAdam, inventor of the paving process, as one of the seven wonders of the modern world: "The Colossus of Roads.")

But his sanguine spirit served him well during the years of war. Despite his ill-met trip to the field to collect his wounded son, despite the deaths of many of his former students, he remained a convinced patriot and propagandist for the Union cause. Lincoln's Democratic opponents thought the doctor a bit laughable and his son was sometimes embarrassed by his father's armchair militancy. On September 13, 1863, Henry Livermore Abbot, a Copperhead comrade of young Holmes, reported home his battlefield opinion that young Captain Holmes "is a student rather than a man of action." He added, "His father, of course, one can't help despising." That sentiment was not surprising in a family of Copperheads. One week after the Emancipation Proclamation, Abbot had written home, "The president's proclamation is of course received with universal disgust, particularly the part which enjoins officers to see that it is carried out." Dr. Holmes had earned such enemies well. He responded to them in his own good-natured way in *The Autocrat of the Breakfast Table*:

"If a fellow attacked my opinions in print, would I reply?" asks the Autocrat. "Not I. Do you think I don't understand what my friend, the Professor, long ago called the hydrostatic paradox of controversy?"—which enigmatic phrase he explained thus: "If you had a bent tube, one arm of which was the size of a pipe-stem and the other big enough to hold the ocean, water would stand at the same height in one as in the other. Thus discussion equalizes fools and wise men in the same way, and the fools know it."

The Autocrat's sanguine temperament also protected him from the Jamesian postwar failure of nerve. He remained as skeptical as before Fort Sumter and maintained the upbeat conviction that folly would by and large yield to reason. When next he came to New York he took aim at an opponent that had not surrendered at Appomattox, quackery. Dr. Holmes appeared before the graduating class of the Bellevue Hospital Medical College in 1871. He began his talk by explaining the difference between the junior and senior members of the profession: the young doctor knows the rules, the older doctor knows the exceptions. He went on to warn the young graduates against the nostrums and "specifics" that passed for therapy in their century. Holmes's next targets were homeopathy, bleeding, and cupping. He advised the young physician to beware the homeopath and his clients:

Some of you will probably be more or less troubled by that parody of medieval theology which finds its dogma in the doctrine of homeopathy, its miracle of transubstantiation in the mystery of its dilutions, its church in the people who have mistaken their century, and its priests in those who have mistaken their calling. You can do little with persons who are disposed to accept these curious medical superstitions. There are those whose minds are satisfied with the million-fold dilution of a scientific proof. No wonder they believe in the efficacy of a similar attenuation of herbs or potions. You have no fulcrum you can rest upon to lift an error out of such minds as these, often highly endowed with knowledge and talent, sometimes with genius, but commonly richer in the imaginative than the observing and reasoning faculties.

His major message was a stern warning that heroic measures, overdosing, and mineral purges were foolish ways of treating disease. He told the students of a surefire cure for agues and rheumatism, a cure safer than purges or bleeding. He advised them to pare the patient's nails, put the parings in a little bag, and hang the bag around the neck of a live eel, and place him in a tub of water. "The eel will die and the patient will recover." This was an extension of the message Holmes had been reading to medical audiences since his manifesto at the Massachusetts Medical Society in 1860: "Throw out opium, which the Creator himself seems to prescribe . . . throw out wine, which is a food, and the vapors which produce the miracle of anesthesia, and I firmly believe that if the whole materia medica, as now used, could be sunk to the bottom—it would be the better for mankind and all the worse for the fishes."

Ever since doctors raised blisters, plied cauteries, and overdosed cases of what they called spinal irritation with calomel, the compliance of foolish patients has been exceeded only by the zeal of foolish physicians. Overuse of calomel, the cortisone of the nineteenth century, had led Holmes to believe that the French were in advance of the English and Americans in the art of prescribing for the sick without hurting them. He far preferred their varied tisanes and syrups to what he called the mineral regimen of bug poison and ratsbane, so long in favor on the other side of the Channel, much as he preferred French cuisine to the "rude cookery of those hard-feeding and much-dosing islanders." He asked whether calomel was not sometimes given by a physician on the same principle by which a landlord occasionally prescribes bacon and eggs, because he could not think of anything else quite so handy.

✳

If calomel was the most overprescribed drug of the nineteenth century, spinal irritation was its most overdiagnosed illness. "Some shrewd old doctors," Dr. Holmes told the Bellevue students, "have a few phrases always on hand for patients who will insist on knowing the pathology of their complaints. . . . I have known the term 'spinal irritation' to serve well on such occasions." It had already served well for over half a century.

The spine became a locus for general malaise in 1821. Dr. R. P. Player of Mansbury reported that when he pressed on certain vertebrae, patients reported pain and were often surprised at the discovery of tenderness in one or another part, the implication of which in disease they had never suspected. But the first complete account of spinal irritation was given in 1828 by one Dr. Thomas Brown of Glasgow. While the spine was at the root of the problem, so to speak, the symptoms were often expressed elsewhere. Some of Dr. Brown's female patients displayed painful, tender spots (beneath the breast or under the sternum) of which they had not been aware until the examination. The morbid sensibility was chiefly in the skin: "The patient for the most part flinches more when the skin is even slightly pinched than when pressure is made on the vertebrae themselves. The pain is in the majority of cases more severe than in those of real vertebral diseases."

Spinal irritation crossed the Atlantic quicker than the submarine cable. At one time or another, most of the eminent Bostonians had their turn. As the male Yankees were off to their countinghouses the malady became practically epidemic among the city's well-off ladies. The generic "madwoman in the attic" of nineteenth-century literature was given calomel or laudanum for spinal trouble. She tended to stay in the attic or a daybed for life, or until the end of the book. Spinal irritation was the excuse for ever more heroic therapy on the part of medical practitioners. Holmes reminded the young students that persons who seek the aid of a physician are very honest and sincere in their wish to get rid of their complaints, because they want to live as long as they can. But since they are desperate to stay alive at any cost,

> there is nothing men will not do, there is nothing they have not done, to recover their health and save their lives. They have submitted to be half-drowned in water, and half-choked with gases, to be buried up to their chins in earth, to be seared with hot irons like galley-slaves, to be crimped with knives, like cod-fish, to have needles thrust into their flesh, and bonfires kindled on their skin, to swallow all sorts of abominations, and to pay for all this, as if to be singed and scalded were a costly privilege, as if blisters were a blessing, and leeches were a luxury.

The great majority of patients subjected to singeing and scalding, to cupping and leeching for aches and pains of the spine, turned out to be women. This folly persists today: A review of recent textbooks and journal articles documents that women constitute between 85 and 95 percent of sufferers from the same symptoms that were once ascribed to "spinal irritations"; in the late twentieth century the ailments are called fibromyalgia, total food allergy, and chronic fatigue syndrome. A history of what passes as psychosomatic disease confirms the notion, tawdry but true, that women in pain are everywhere hassled by men with promises. One need not be a feminist critic to trace the foolish practices of today to their roots in medical misogyny. History teaches us that social norms shape medical fashion and that medical fashion in turn shapes the symptoms that patients select. A prominent historian of medicine, Edward Shorter, suggests in his *From Paralysis to Fatigue* (1992) that "most of the symptoms of psychosomatic disease have always been known to Western society, although they have occurred at different times with different frequencies: Society does not invent symptoms; it retrieves them from the symptom pool."

As was the case with spinal irritation, many patients with fibromyalgia or chronic fatigue syndrome are no doubt afflicted by an as yet obscure response to chemicals or viruses; new candidates propose themselves weekly. But real microbes eventually cause diseases that really hurt, that kill, maim, or provoke detectable bodily ill. That's not the point of the psychosomatic argument. "The unconscious mind," our historian tells us, "desires to be taken seriously and not be ridiculed. It will therefore strive to present symptoms that always seem, to the surrounding culture, legitimate evidence of organic disease." The patient must present symptoms that the medical culture cannot reject. By hook or by crook, by stealth or by wealth, new symptoms arise that evade the doctor's new gadgets.

✳

The diagnosis of spinal irritation and its treatment by counterirritation reached its zenith in the 1886 book *Spinal Irritation*, by Dr. W. A. Hammond of New York. He routinely found "multiple tender spots" in women suffering from spinal irritation and ascribed some of the cases to sexual excess or, so he was convinced, masturbation. In keeping with his contemporaries, he advocated treatment with "counterirritants" such as dry heat, scalding water, or croton oil extracts. William Alexander Hammond had been for a short time Surgeon General of the United States. He attained the distinction, unique for that rank, of being court-martialed during the Civil War after acrimonious squabbles with Secretary of War Stanton and bureaucrats of the career Medical Service. His chief problem, aside from a personal lapse in petty finance, seems to have been that he was too closely affiliated with the reformers of the Sanitary Commission.

But Hammond was able to recover from political infamy; eventually his reputation was cleansed and his rank restored by the Senate. He went on to become one of the founders not only of the American Neurological Association but also of the NYU Postgraduate Medical School, in the library of which his books are now quietly disintegrating. Hammond's magisterial *A Treatise on Diseases of the Nervous System* (1871), the first American textbook of neurology, is an extensive tome, published a scant seven years after his fall from official grace. The treatise is filled with outmoded rituals and jawbreaking syndromes. Scattered among this dross are neatly described case histories and new observations, but the volume is tough slogging.

In contrast, Hammond's other professorial book, *A Treatise on Insanity in Its Medical Relations* (1883), is only 738 pages long and can be read like fiction—the stuff of Maupassant or William Dean Howells. The chapters on "hysteria" and "hypochondriacal mania" yield the richest lode of stories. Hammond's characters include Eliza C, "who crowned herself with flowers, took a guitar, and announced that she was going to travel through the world. She got up in the night and washed her clothes in the chamber-pot. Then she had convulsions, mewed like a cat, tried to climb up the wall and finally fell into a state of stupor." Brief, mad lives are recounted by the hundreds in this astounding compendium, including astute Colonel Charles May of the U.S. Army, who—by means of bloodless, bogus surgery—cured a fellow officer "of the belief that he was inhabited by chicken bones."

Poor Miss A.W., a patient of Hammond's, had the habit of swallowing pins by the dozen. She later extruded these pins from her skin, her nose, and various nether orifices (surely the first documented case of pins envy). We also learn of a "young lady from a Western city" who had "grasped a large knife that lay on the table and would have killed her mother with it had it not been seized by her sister, who was present." She explained this subsequently by saying that she had thought her mother "was a black man who was stealing her jewelry."

Hammond shows warmth and empathy for his mentally ill patients, regarding them in the tolerant, bemused fashion of a Victorian author displaying his fictional creatures:

> Kindness and forbearance, supported by firmness, will not altogether fail in their influence with even the most confirmed and degraded lunatics. Probably the most difficult class of patients to manage by moral means is that of the reasoning maniacs, and next to them those cases of hysterical mania which exhibit marked perversities of character and disposition. But even with such people the principles of justice and fair dealing will not be lost, and eventually an impression will probably be made on subjects incapable of being touched by other measures.

But woe to the patient who failed to respond to "moral means," the talking cure. She—for it was usually a female patient—was in for leeches or counterirritants:

> On the other hand, local bloodletting by cups or leeches is often a useful measure, especially in those cases in which there are pain and heat in the head accompanied with insomnia and excitement. A couple of leeches to the inside of the nostrils are remarkably efficacious in relieving cerebral hyperaemia [too much blood in the brain] and mitigating the violence of the physical and mental symptoms resulting from it. As to counter-irritants, such as blisters, croton oil, tartarized antimony, and the actual cautery, cases every now and then appear in which they seem to be of service. I have, however, several times aggravated the mental and physical symptoms of insanity by their use. I suppose the most generally advantageous agent of the kind is the actual cautery very lightly

applied to the nucha [the back of the neck], but then the action in such a case can scarcely be called counter-irritant.

For simple hysteria, talking cures seem to work best, and it mattered not which learned profession did the talking or listening. A young lady twenty years of age began to wear "pads over the abdomen and gradually increased their thickness" until, confronted by her parents, she confessed to unwed pregnancy and declared a gentleman lawyer they all knew and respected to be her seducer. The outraged father offered the barrister the alternative of "an immediate marriage or instant death from a pistol pointed at his head . . . the pistol, cocked, was very near his brain." Only after he had unwillingly agreed to this handgun marriage did the lawyer have a chance to chat with his betrothed. Using measures less severe than leeches or cautery, the lawyer by his tact and the directness of his questions succeeded in exposing the fraud and obtaining a full confession. The marriage was canceled and Hammond was engaged to complete the cure.

Some of these human vignettes can be read as drafts for the melodramatic or Gothic novels of Hammond's day; in this context, Dr. Holmes's *Elsie Venner* comes to mind. But the anecdotes were intended to reveal neither the character of individuals nor the nature of the society in which they moved. Instead, only enough detail was given to illustrate the variegated clinical forms of hysteria or spinal irritation.

Spinal irritation or inflammation eventually became the basis of an organized religion: Christian Science. Mary Baker Glover Patterson Eddy suffered a small epiphany when she hurt her back in 1866. Her injury was an obscure hurt that seemed to mimic that of Henry James the younger. She was literally struck by the notion that since "matter and death are mortal illusions," one could overcome disease by exercise of mind. There is, in fact, a large area of agreement between this notion and those expressed by James the elder in *Shadow and Substance*. What a Bostonian affliction! Poor Mary Baker Eddy was troubled all her life by "spinal inflammation and its train of suffering—gastric and bilious" to the point where her second husband had to carry her downstairs for her wedding ceremony—and back to her invalid bed directly thereafter. Sure enough, with the help of healing and the mind, she was soon able to climb all 182 steps of Portland's city hall tower. Eddy and her followers were persuaded that Christian Science and its healers constituted the main line of defense against "malicious animal magnetism," which was the main cause of illness and death. This not unpersuasive system of alternative medicine has continued to outlast its origins in spinal irritation.

As the last century wound down, rational France was again swept by medical unreason. Spinal irritation yielded to "hysteria" under the careful ministrations of Jean Martin Charcot (1825–93). Charcot began his career as an astute internist and his clinical observations remain part of the literature of modern medicine. But once he turned to diseases of the mind, he became a Barnum of the mental wards. These days he is regarded as little more than a link between Mesmer and Freud. As with Agassiz, most observers agree in retrospect that there was more humbug than matter to his theory; if his talents were clinical, his genius was theatrical. Charcot's clinical demonstrations at the Salpêtrière were open to the public, and a generation of dazed, sick women were displayed to an audience of fashionable voyeurs. The sessions were in stiff competition with the boulevard theaters of the *fin de siècle*, and perhaps for that reason most of the clinical syndromes Charcot described, such as *grande hystérie*, are now believed to have been either fancied or staged.

A student of Charcot, Dr. Jean-Albert Pitres of Bordeaux, found that attacks of *grande hystérie* took their origin in—you might have guessed—certain tender spots. In cases of hysteria,

Dr. Pitres was able to define a "demarcated spasmogenic zone" over his patients' bodies (the small of the back, both armpits, and the bottom of the sternum) as well as over the ovary.

Sigmund Freud, who had traveled to the Salpêtrière to sit at Charcot's feet, was also a devotee of the tender-spot doctrine. He described hysteria in terms that might astound not only feminists. His patient Fräulein Elizabeth von R. had such an area, and when Freud touched a sensitive spot on her skin, she cried out. He could not help thinking that it was as though she were "having a voluptuous tickling sensation; her face flushed, she threw back her head and shut her eyes and her body bent backwards." Another of Freud's patients, Frau K., had in 1895 cramplike pains in her chest. "In her case," Freud told his friend Wilhelm Fliess in 1895, "I have invented a strange therapy of my own: I search for sensitive areas, press on them, and thus provoke fits of shaking which free her." His patient's spasmogenic zones, originally in her face, shifted to two points on her left chest wall—identical, Freud said, to his own spasmogenic points. But before we rush Freud to the wall for what we know to be the *real* meaning of all this, we might recall that the method we use to arrive at our conclusions was devised by him.

The remedy for all those myalgias, for all that accumulated pain and fatigue, was a century-long, concentrated attack by male doctors on the female reproductive tract. More than half of the articles dealing with oophorectomy in 1889 described it as a treatment for mental disease; hysteria (from the Greek word for womb) has, of course, been traditionally attributed to disorders of the womb or ovaries. Other modes of therapy for spinal irritation or hysteria included cauterization of the clitoris, hysterectomy, curettage, cupping, electroshock, and arsenic.

But the diagnostic fancies of pressure points and tender spots followed by counterirritants and nostrums are not limited to the past. The folly persists today, as can be seen from the fibromyalgia literature. The presence of eleven or more of eighteen "specific tender point sites" together with widespread pain in the *absence* of radiographic or lab abnormalities, suffices now-adays for the official classification of fibromyalgia. Doctors who believe in this diagnosis today elicit pain at the magic spots of their mainly female patients by means of either a pain-metering machine or "palpation with the pulp of the thumb or the first 2 or 3 fingers at a pressure of approximately 4 kilos." One text-book expert of the 1990s suggests a variety of treatments for this syndrome under the general rubric "Counterirritant Therapy." These include "a wide variety of popular or unusual therapies, including massage, heat, liniments, steroid injections, ethyl chloride spray, and acupuncture," all of which he believes to be helpful in relieving pain and which sound very much like Hammond's prescriptions for spinal irritation. Since the magic potions haven't changed for over a century we might call this cult medicine, rather than science. Our expert confirms that notion: "Factors influencing a choice of counterirritant technique will include simplicity, safety, and availability and economy on one hand and maximal placebo effect on the other."

Women, and not men, will be subject to these measures for the therapy not only of fibromyalgia but also "irritable bowel" and "chronic fatigue syndrome," the official criteria for which differ very slightly from those for fibromyalgia. One might therefore ask whether sexism, historical folly, or medical science is at work; homeopathy and its kindred delusions revisited, we might answer.

The world of Holmes and the black-bag doctors whom he addressed seems far away, viewed from our privileged decade of molecular medicine, of sono- and angiograms, of cyclo- and cephalosporins, of liposomes and liposuction. The day-to-day medicine of the 1830s–1930s appears to have been futile, groping—let's face it, *quackish.* All that laying on of hands, thumping of the chest, calomel, glycerine, cautery, compresses! Nevertheless, Holmes gave the young Bellevue physicians a me-liorist vision of the medical profession which transcends the fashionable diagnoses and drugs of the day; it will remain true when colonoscopy will have gone the way of cautery, and cortisone the way of calomel:

> If the cinchona trees all died out . . . and the arsenic mines were exhausted, and the sulphur regions were burned up, if every drug from the vegetable, animal, and mineral kingdom were to disappear from the market, a body of enlightened men, organized as a distinct profession, would be required just as much as now, and respected and trusted as now, whose province should be to guard against the causes of disease, to eliminate them if possible when still present, to order all the conditions of the patient so as to favor the efforts of the system to right itself, and to give those predictions of the course of disease which only experience can warrant, and which in so many cases relieve the exaggerated fears of sufferers and their friends, or warn them in season of impending danger. Great as the loss would be if certain active remedies could no longer be obtained, it would leave the medical profession the most essential part of its duties, and all, and more than all, its present share of *honor.*

III. THE FLOWERING OF DNA

In this world our colossal immodesty
has plundered and poisoned, it is possible
  You still might save us, who by now have
  learned this: that scientists, to be truthful,

must remind us to take all they say as a
tall story, that abhorred in the Heav'ns are all
  self-proclaimed poets who, to wow an
  audience, utter some resonant lie.

  —W. H. Auden, "Ode to Terminus," 1966

11. ALICE JAMES AND NEUROTIC SCIENCE

I am being ground slowly on the grim grindstone of physical pain and on two nights I had almost asked for K's lethal dose, but one steps hesitatingly along unaccustomed ways and endures from second to second. . . .

—Alice James, *Journal*, March 4, 1892

The lethal dose would have been laudanum, and the "K" who dispensed it would have been Alice James's faithful companion, Katherine Peabody Loring. A few days after she wrote this entry Alice James was dead from metastatic cancer, killed by what she called "this unholy granite substance in my breast." Better known today than in her lifetime, the younger sister of Henry and William James took to her bed many years before her fatal disease. Nowadays, her lifelong invalidism might be called fibromyalgia, chronic fatigue syndrome, conversion hysteria, or somatization reaction. In her day it was called "a gouty diathesis," "spinal neurosis," "nervous hyperaesthesia," or "neurasthenia." Our names and medicines for these complaints have not improved much. Alice James knew that she was not physically ill in any real sense and awaited the rise of "neurotic science." She was treated by the most eminent physicians of her time with Indian hemp (cannabis), galvanic stimulation, and a variety of water cures. Then cancer struck. On May 31, 1891, she wrote:

To him who waits, all things come! My aspirations have been
eccentric, but I cannot complain now that they have not been
brilliantly fulfilled. Ever since I have been ill, I have longed
and longed for some palpable disease, no matter how conven-
tionally dreadful a label it might have . . . It is entirely inde-
cent to catalogue one's self in this way, but I put it down in
a scientific spirit, to show that though I have no productive
worth, I have a certain value as an indestructible quantity.

Indestructible she was not, but she continued nevertheless to
produce in her journal an indestructible work of literature that
ranks with those of her brothers. It is a record of daily events,
an almanac that condenses a decade, and a sharp text of self-
knowledge. It had begun simply enough, in an English spa to
which she had retreated for the waters: "Leamington, May,
1889. I think that if I get into the habit of writing a bit about
what happens, or rather doesn't happen, I may lose a little of
the sense of loneliness and despair which abides by me." But
soon she found her own style, in which social insight, cutting
wit, and a good nose for literature mixed well with a bent for
Reform, a tendency to what brother Henry called "passionate
radicalism." She was a sharp critic of conservative politics; a fan
of Irish Home Rule and Parnell; she was also ahead of her time
in sniffing out the cost of empire. She worried about an English
class structure in which:

. . . the working man allows himself to be patted and legislated
out of all independence; thus the profound ineradicables in
the bone and the sinew conviction that outlying regions are
their preserves, that they alone of human races massacre sav-
ages out of pure virtue. It would ill become an American to
reflect upon the treatment of aboriginal races; but I never
heard it suggested that our hideous dealings with the Indians
was brotherly love under the guise of pure cussedness.

After her tumor was diagnosed, the tone of her journal turned somewhat darker and the entries more confessional. She permitted herself at last to express deep love for her long-term companion, Katherine Loring, producing passages that recall the yellow clovers of Katharine Lee Bates: "In lieu of words too grievous to be spoken." Loring was a competent, educated woman of Brahmin stock, of whom Alice James had written to Sara Darwin (Charles Darwin's American daughter-in-law): "She has all the mere brute superiority which distinguishes man from woman combined with all the distinctively feminine virtues. There is nothing she cannot do from hewing wood and drawing water to driving run-away horses & educating all the women in North America." Late pictures show her as a tidy, angular individual: Alice B. Toklas as nurse-confidante. An incisive sketch by John Singer Sargent of the two Loring sisters shows two purposeful creatures living in sunlight and shadow.

Katherine Loring had given up an active life to be with Alice James, shuttling between her consumptive sister and the intermittently paralyzed James. In the last few months of her life, the journal was no longer written by Alice James herself, but dictated to K. Alice James's tribute at what she called "this mortuary moment" is therefore perhaps more poignant:

> . . . is it not wonderful that this unholy granite substance in my breast should be the soil propitious for the perfect flowering of Katherine's unexampled genius for friendship and devotion. The story of her watchfulness, patience, and untiring resource, cannot be told by my feeble pen, but the pain and discomfort seem a feeble price to pay for all the happiness and peace with which she fills my days.

Alice James contrasted the devotion of her friend with the more distant attention paid by her attending physicians. Sir Andrew Clarke is reprimanded for never quite being on time: he is of course the *late* Sir Andrew. But the eminent cancer specialist cannot help her; she is afraid that he is gripped by "impotent paralysis" and "talking by the hour without *saying* anything, while the longing, pallid victim stretches out a sickly tendril, hoping for some excrescence, a human wart, to catch on to." Alice James then utters a cry from Keats's world of pains and troubles: "When will men pass from the illusion of the intellectual, limited to sapless reason, and bow to the intelligent, juicy with the succulent science of life?"

The science of life, biology, ought in some way to be able to account not only for how tumor suppressor genes influence breast cancer but also for the lifelong affliction of souls as fragile as Alice James. The most convenient biological explanation is a genetic one, and keepers of the Jamesian flame point to a striking cluster of nervous pathology in two generations of the family. Deep depression, hysterical paralyses, and sexual ambiguity seemed to run in the clan: father Henry suffered from his Swedenborgian "midnight vastation," Henry, Jr., ran into the obscure hurt of his "dorsal anguish" on the day of Fort Sumter, William was paralyzed by "quivering fear" in the course of his own vastation. Mental homes provided refuge for the "incommunicable sadness" of youngest brother Rob and the "madness" of cousin Kitty. Alice herself retreated to the Adams Nervine Asylum.

William James, loftiest of the brood, believed that the Jameses literally carried a genetic load on their back. Using the imagery of spinal irritation, he wrote Rob, "I account it as a true crime against humanity for any one to run the probable risk of generating unhealthy offspring. For myself I have long since fully determined never to marry with anyone . . . for this dorsal trouble is evidently s'thing in the blood."

But social explanations rival the genetic. In her remarkable biography, *Alice James* (1980), Jean Strouse has argued plausibly that Alice James's flight into disease was at least in part a not uncommon female strategy for coping with oppressive male society in general and her father's expectations specifically. Strouse attributes some of Alice's symptoms to a daughter's reaction to a "kind father who had so blithely stimulated and thwarted her." She calls attention to Alice James's recollection of an acute early episode:

> As I used to sit immovable reading in the library with waves of violent inclination suddenly invading my muscles taking some one of their myriad forms such as throwing myself out of the window, or *knocking off the head of the benignant pater* as he sat with his silver locks, writing at his table, it used to seem to me that the only difference between me and the insane was that I had not only all the horrors and suffering of insanity but the duties of doctor, nurse and strait-jacket imposed upon me, too. [italics added]

The words drop on the page like nuggets of Strindberg—or Freud. But, in retrospect, no one can blame with confidence either nature or nurture for Alice James's life of infirmity, for her unasked-for crucifixion, to use a phrase of Oliver Sacks's. Nurture in the form of nineteenth-century medical practice was clearly responsible for the diagnoses pinned on Alice James in her lifetime: spinal irritation, neurasthenia, hysteria, suppressed gout, etc. Medical practice was also responsible for subjecting her to electric prods, Indian hemp, spinal manipulation, and those innumerable buckets of tepid spa water, "as if to be singed and scalded were a costly privilege and leeches were a luxury," à la Dr. Holmes.

Alice was one of many poor spirits who were flogged from pillar to post on the premise that their paralyses and palpitations were due to rebel humors in the spine. A routine case of "nervous affliction of the spine," she would not have earned a footnote in Dr. Hammond's treatise. But the crude treatments she underwent were not simply due to the general assault of male doctors on their spinally challenged female patients. The male version of hysteria was called hypochondriasis and the paralyses it produced were also, willy-nilly, attributed to spinal irritation. Fresh from the Harvard Medical School, William James advised the most nervous of the James brothers, Rob, to "take iron, to exercise, and to apply enough iodine to your back until the skin peels." Shades of Dr. Hammond's counterirritation! In the end, her mother, Mary, knew what was wrong with Alice James, correctly judging that "it is a case of genuine hysteria for which no cause as yet can be discovered."

A century later, we are not much further along in solving the puzzle of hysteria. Sad to say, and despite the remarkable progress we have made in the molecular biology of oncogenes, we're not much further along with breast cancer either. In the hundred years since Alice James suffered from one and died from the other of these ailments, we know somewhat more about the epidemiology of mental disease and have gotten better at the surgery of breast cancer, but their chemistry still escapes us. The science of life, succulent or not, still has a long way to go.

Alice James's journal of disease and despair brings a tableau to mind. It is set in a Kensington drawing room that might have been painted by John Singer Sargent, but the feeling is pure Edvard Munch. It is January 6, 1892, and Alice has just finished reading Emily Dickinson's poems, posthumously collected by Colonel Thomas Wentworth Higginson. It is two months before her death and she is racked by the jaundice of liver metastases. A photograph taken at the time shows Alice in her daybed; she looks drawn and gaunt, but has been dressed up and beribboned for the photographer. She sits stiffly propped on her cushions and appears pain-free for a while on morphine: the poppy is singing its song. She can no longer concentrate enough to write and dictates her journal entries to the beloved K. But K is by no means the only reader for whom the *pensées* are intended; Alice is also leaving a record for her brothers William and

Henry. Her last letter to William pleads, ". . . when I'm gone, pray don't think of me simply as a creature who might have been something else, had neurotic science been born."

Emily Dickinson has struck a chord in that sickroom. Indeed, Dickinson's is the *only* poem in English to be found in Alice James's journal. But the subject of her journal entry on January 6 isn't only death, and it isn't only Emily Dickinson and it certainly isn't Colonel Higginson, undervalued as always by his loftier readers. No, the subject is the family serpent, and it is no accident that she is reminded of her last visit from a Darwin:

> It is reassuring to hear the English pronouncement that Emily Dickinson is fifth-rate—they have such a capacity for missing quality; the robust evades them equally with the subtle. Her being sicklied o'er with T. W. Higginson makes one quake lest there be a latent flaw which escapes one's vision; but what tomes of philosophy *resume* the cheap farce, or express the highest point of view of the aspiring soul more completely than the following:
>
> > *How dreary to be somebody;*
> > *How public, like a frog,*
> > *To tell your name the livelong day*
> > *To an admiring bog!*

Alice James connects Dickinson to her own fate via Mesmer. "Dr. Tuckey [a Mesmeric doctor] asked me the other day whether I had written for the press. I vehemently denied the imputation. How sad it is that the purely innocuous should always be supposed to have the trail of the family serpent upon them."

The family serpent is, of course, the double helix of depression and inspiration that ran through the James family, that "dorsal trouble . . . in the blood." Indeed, immediately after quoting the Dickinson poem, Alice James dictates an account of a visit paid her years before by Charles Darwin's daughter, Henrietta Litchfield. When Alice James told Mrs. Litchfield that her invalidism had for years been called "latent gout," the Darwin lady exclaimed, "Oh! that's what we have [in our family], does it come from drink in your parents?" The Darwins, like the Jameses, were a clan of morose geniuses, scholars and medics who also seem to have had a family serpent in the blood. The Darwin biographies document a strong family history of depression, somatization reactions, and wives who took to their beds for decades. Sure enough, much of this pathology was blamed on spinal irritation, or a "gouty diathesis." Depression and inspiration were closely intertwined in the Darwin line, as closely—one might say—as the two dancing serpents on the crest of Darwin College, Cambridge.

❋

The one serpent that certainly did *not* run in the blood of either family was gout. A point of irony will attract the medical reader of Alice James's journal at this point, for it turns out that one of the few physicians who told her exactly what was wrong with her and who explained that gout had little to do with her lifelong infirmity was Sir Alfred Baring Garrod (1819–1907), the Darwin of gout. Alice James reported that she had "spent the most affable hour of my life" with Garrod, who told her in 1884 that the weakness in her legs and her digestive complaints were functional and not "organic." But—as usual with her doctors—she soon became disenchanted. At the dawn of the Freudian age she complained:

> I could get nothing out of him & he slipped thro' my cramped & clinging grasp as skillfully as if his physical conformation had been that of an eel instead of a Dutch cheese. The gout he looks upon as a small part of my trouble, 'it being complicated with an excessive nervous sensibility,' but I could get no suggestions of any sort as to climate, baths, or diet from

him. The truth was he was entirely puzzled about me and had
not the manliness to say so.

Whether like an eel or a Dutch cheese in manly conformation,
Garrod no less than Darwin is one of the ancestors of modern
molecular genetics. For A. B. Garrod, in *The Nature and Treatment of Gout and Rheumatic Gout* (1859), was the first not only
to show that excess uric acid in the blood was invariably associated with gout, but also to distinguish between the heritable
and more epidemic form of gout—saturnine gout—a disease
which had been rampant in the ruling classes of England since
the eighteenth century and which is caused by drinking fortified
wine.

The story of saturnine gout is more than a simple tale of how
the ingestion of lead produces the features of gout: acute ar-
thritis, chalky deposits on the joints (tophi), and kidney disease.
In its own way, it is a social comedy of table manners. In an
effort to stem the tide, as it were, of French wine imports, the
English Foreign Minister, Methuen, signed a treaty with Portugal in 1703 which permitted fortified wine (port and Madeira)
to be imported from Portugal at a fraction of the cost of the
French products. He had simultaneously struck a blow to
French exports and English kidneys. Wines such as port, Madeira, and Malaga are "fortified" by adding distilled alcohol or
brandy. But the stills of the Portuguese in the eighteenth century
ground exceedingly fine: they were lined, or joined, by lead.
Lead leached from the stills found its way into the finished
product and remained in the bottle until drunk. The alcohol was
added to fortified wine not only to give it more kick but to
prevent spoilage and deterioration on storage. It worked: the
port lasted, and the lead remained. Indeed, recent spectroscopic
analyses of rare eighteenth-century fortified wine—on sale at
Christie's—showed them to contain 1,900 micrograms per liter
as opposed to the 180 micrograms per liter found in their
present-day counterparts.

In the event, by 1825 the English were importing 40,277 tuns (1 tun = 252 old wine gallons) of fortified wine each year. The colonies, too, did their part, until the war of 1812 stopped the overflow (so to speak) to American shores. The disease in England and the colonies took its greatest toll among the middle and upper classes, for the poor drank mainly gin and beer. The well-off drank fortified wine and became fit subjects for cartoonists who lampooned the ruby-nosed and red-footed gentry lapsing into tophi and tremors. Neither the French nobility, who quaffed their lead-free burgundy or claret straight, nor Scottish lairds, who made do with whiskey, had a like incidence of gout. Since the epidemic of saturnine gout was due to nurture, not nature, Garrod and his contemporaries had a good notion of what to do: they sent their well-off patients to Bath or Leamington, expecting that a few weeks of the water cure would flush the metal from their system. Nowadays, we are confronted with saturnine gout of another sort: the moonshine gout of the rural South or the Mexican border. Here the distillation vessel is likely to be an old radiator or pottery decorated with lead paint, but the offending metal is still the same.

But why is lead-induced gout called "saturnine"? In alchemical notation, lead was the sign of Saturn, farthest away and slowest of all the planets. Astrologers believed, and nowadays alternative medical folks *still* believe, that those born under the sign of Saturn are cold, sluggish, and morose of temperament; depressed, as it were. But after the eighteenth century, notions of a morose temperament became joined to the gentlemanly ideal of gravity (*gravitas*) and of rank; the saturnine peerage spent over a century "drunk as lords" on lead-laced port. At the noble feast in Keats's "Lamia," for example, "wine came from a gloomy tun." It is no accident that gravitas, depression, and "a gouty diathesis" came to be linked in the popular and medical mind with the drinking habits of the gentry. And by the time Garrod attended Alice James, "the honor of the gout" had been extended to the intellectually gifted and morose. With lead as the metallic culprit, the saturnine Jameses and Darwins were in their proper element, so to speak.

Disentangling the saturnine from heritable forms of gout was a neat solution to a tough riddle of nature and nurture; and Dr. Garrod deserves full marks. Indeed, those who study the molecular basis of gout can argue that George Eliot was perhaps too quick to scold Lydgate for abandoning science to "write a treatise on gout, a disease which has a good deal of wealth on its side." In point of fact, Garrod's treatise on gout had consequences as large as those produced by Eliot's real-life heroes, Bichat and Louis. Garrod's "string sign," which was used to show high levels of uric acid in the blood of the gouty and their families, was the beginning of modern biochemical genetics.

Garrod left us yet another legacy. His son Sir Archibald Edward Garrod followed his father's lead on the heritable nature of gout. He became interested in a series of rare genetic disorders which he called "inborn errors of metabolism" (1908). And it is thanks to modern studies of inborn errors of metabolism—phenylketonuria is a prime example—that the principle emerged of "one gene, one enzyme." By means of that principle, François Jacob and Jacques Monod were able in 1961 to discover how changes in nutrients *outside* a bacterium can switch single genes on or off *within* the cell; an example of how nurture modifies nature in the dish. Nowadays, when we treat phenylketonurics by means of an appropriate diet from birth, we can prevent both physical and mental disease; this is a striking example of how nurture can modify nature in the clinic as well. Clues from the study of depression suggest that the family serpent of gloom in the blood may also turn out to be an inborn error of metabolism. The irony would not have escaped either William or Alice James that the Garrods, who began the science of gout, were present at the birth of "neurotic science."

✳

The case can be made that the resonance between Alice James (1848–92) and Emily Dickinson (1830–86) relates less to the genetics of family mood than to the Puritan culture to which they were heir. Diana Trilling has linked the lives of these two depressed and inspired spinsters, tucked away in their collective hundred years of solitude. The summary from Morningside Heights seems fair enough: "Alice James and Emily Dickinson," she wrote in 1947, "protested the life of public recognition too violently, just as each of them inevitably demanded, in what she sent into the world, too much attention for *herself*, but it is a common failing among women of talent."

Instructed by Sacvan Bercovitch's scholarly *The Puritan Origins of the American Self*, one might add that this interplay between private needs and public demands is not limited to *women* of talent. Drawing on the examples of Emerson and Whitman, Bercovitch argues that the Puritan ethos produced in some American artists, men no less than women, the need to create a country of one's self, to write an "auto-American-biography" in which "the private state no less than the public is manifest destiny." And of Emerson's darker moods, Bercovitch writes, "To despair in oneself is a symbolic gesture of equal magnitude to the affirmation of the national dream." In this view, God's work on earth can also be done in the private sphere. Governor Winthrop's city on the hill—or Katharine Lee Bates's alabaster city, for that matter—has an internal surrogate in the Puritan soul. But those alabaster cities of the mind are oft dim'd by human tears.

Emily Dickinson's verse at the deathbed of Alice James suggests that the Dickinson version of auto-American-biography differs very much from that of Emerson or Whitman. "I hear America singing," chants Whitman. "I hear America sobbing," sighs Emily Dickinson. One is reminded that great poets are more likely to be depressed than elated, loners than joiners, patients than doctors. Like the journal of Alice James, the poems of Emily Dickinson constitute an auto-American-biography.

But the life recounted is that of a patient—any patient—looking
for a doctor with time enough to listen "while the longing, pallid
victim stretches out a sickly tendril." That victim, had she the
voice, might imagine her last moments like this:

> *I heard a Fly buzz—when I died—*
> *The Stillness in the Room*
> *Was like the Stillness in the Air*
> *Between the Heaves of Storm—* . . .
> *With blue—uncertain stumbling buzz—*
> *Between the light—and me—*
> *And then the Windows failed—and then*
> *I could not see to see—*

When Emily Dickinson died of what was diagnosed as
Bright's disease at the age of fifty-five, she left behind an aston-
ishing body of work—almost two thousand poems. Many of
these are the glory of American poetry; they can also be read as
a poignant case history of a woman in pain. Set to a Puritan
hymn beat, or as a wag would have it, to the tune of "The
Yellow Rose of Texas," her lines are trimmed as carefully as
boxwood on the Amherst green. But the poems are neither de-
votional nor inspirational in a conventional mode. They are almost uniformly depressed in sentiment and drop like tears on
the page. Here are some of her opening lines:

> *I felt a Funeral in my Brain*
> *And Mourners to and fro* . . .
>
> *The Soul selects her own Society—*
> *Then—shuts the Door—*
>
> *The Heart asks Pleasure—first—*
> *And then—Excuse from Pain—*
>
> *My life closed twice before its close;*
> *It yet remains to see* . . .

> *Because I could not stop for Death*
> *He kindly stopped for me . . .*

Rarely does Dickinson swing to the other pole of those dark sentiments, but when she does, we get a glimpse of what might have been, had neurotic science been born:

> *Inebriate of Air—am I—*
> *And Debauchee of Dew—*
> *Reeling—thro endless summer days—*
> *From inns of Molten Blue—*

But by and large, the downs have it six-love over the ups: the dew has gone from the grass: "As imperceptibly as Grief / The summer lapsed away . . ." The reader of these lamentations soon realizes he has been permitted into the Society of a very wounded Soul indeed. The poetry has about it the sounds of a patient carefully arranging her symptoms. Clinicians know that the words patients use to describe their aches are carefully, if not always consciously, chosen to evoke specific responses from the doctor: a pill, an injection, a treatment, a warning, some comfort. Above all, the patient wants an open ear and attentive eye, to be received as Alice James was by good doctor Garrod, who "listened with apparent interest and attention to my oft-repeated tale, which by the way to save breath and general exhaustion I am going to have printed in a small pamphlet." In one sense, Alice James's journal and Emily Dickinson's poems are precisely that small pamphlet, a case record from Keats's world of pains and troubles.

What the patient chooses to tell the doctor, the cues that are given, can be compared to what—at the level of art—a poet or writer selects for the reader. Alice reminds one of William James in his psychology lab; her "oft-repeated tale" is the stimulus, the doctor's "interest and attention" are the expected response. That stimulus/response aspect of poetry was proposed by one of the founders of the American Society of Clinical Investigation, Dr. Alfred E. Cohn, then at the Rockefeller Institute. He told an audience at the Metropolitan Museum of Art in 1930 that poetry of Dickinson's sort was "the poet's opportunity to deal exquisitely with human nature . . . it is an experiment as carefully calculated as one in physiology." And the physiology lab he had in mind was that of William James's successor, Walter B. Cannon.

The human nature of Emily Dickinson has been dealt with exquisitely by legions of literati and platoons of psychologists. They seem to agree that her poems fulfill Cohn's criterion: the verse is, indeed, as carefully calculated as an experiment in physiology. They disagree on the point of that experiment, however. Psychoanalytic monographs focus on Emily Dickinson's father or the identity of his surrogates. Feminist critics have cited her attachment to Helen Hunt Jackson and her repressed sexuality: Rebecca Patterson believed she had solved the "riddle of Emily Dickinson," but the late poet laureate, Philip Larkin, echoing Howells, suggests that she kept it.

The English still miss Dickinson's quality. Larkin, a saturnine boozer himself, delivered the verdict from Hull: "If Emily Dickinson could write 700 pages of poems and three volumes of letters without making clear the nature of her preoccupations, then we can be sure that she was determined to keep it hidden . . . and that her inspiration derived in part from keeping it hidden. The price she paid was that of appearing to posterity as perpetually unfinished and wilfully eccentric." But here in America her fans have carried the day, and nowadays she is as much part of the canon as apple pie. In the survey courses she now occupies the midpoint of auto-American-biography between Transcendental Emerson and confessional Robert Lowell.

Emily Dickinson also has a large following in France, where likenesses have been noted between her poetry and that of

Baudelaire, her contemporary. Both poets wrote verse which describes the experience of transcending sickness to a kind of nervous, fragile health. There is, in fact, an exact parallel to Dickinson's "I felt a Funeral in my Brain / And Mourners to and fro" in Baudelaire's *"Et de longs corbillards, sans tambours ni musique / Defilent lentement dans mon âme"* ("Long hearses without drums or music / File in procession through my soul"). Dickinson's "Hope is the thing with Feathers / that perches in the Soul" is an image that resonates with the French *"Où l'Espérance, comme un chauve-souris / S'en va battant les murs de son aile timid"* ("Where Hope, like a bat / beats its timid wings against the wall"). And the mid-nineteenth-century experience of early death from infectious disease or civil insurrection rambles through both their verses. For Dickinson: "A Service, like a Drum— / Kept beating—beating—till I thought / My Mind was going numb . . ." Baudelaire also played with funereal sounds:

> *Vers un cimitière isolé,*
> *Mon coeur comme un tambour voilé*
> *Va battant des marches funèbres.*
>
> *(My heart like a muffled drum*
> *Beats out a funeral march*
> *Toward a lonely cemetery.)*

Mid-nineteenth-century poets loved this metaphor: In "The Psalm of Life," Longfellow's "hearts though stout and brave" also beat "Funeral marches to the grave." "The Grateful Dead" is Dr. William Crosby's inspired title for his translation of one of Baudelaire's funereal rambles, but it could serve that function equally well for a dozen of Emily Dickinson's. Death, who was kind enough to stop for Dickinson, stopped to "plant a flag" on the skull of Charles Baudelaire.

Yet Emily Dickinson was the very opposite of the dark Par-

isian dandy. She was an American rural naif. Colonel Higginson
describes his first meeting with her:

> . . . a step like a pattering child's in entry . . . a little plain
> woman . . . two smooth bands of reddish hair and a face with
> no good feature . . . She came to me with two day-lilies, which
> she put in a sort of childlike way into my hands and said,
> 'These are my introduction,' in a soft, frightened, breathless
> childlike voice—and added under her breath, 'Forgive me
> if I am frightened; I never see strangers, and hardly know
> what I say'—but she talked soon and thence forward
> continuously—and deferentially—sometimes stopping to ask
> me to talk instead of her—but readily recommencing.

Were it not for Higginson, whom we've encountered in South
Carolina with Charlotte Forten, at Faneuil Hall with Samuel
Gridley Howe, and at the Lyceum with Edgar Allan Poe, Dick-
inson might have remained one of Holmes's "Voiceless":

> *A few can touch the magic string,*
> *And noisy Fame is proud to win them:—*
> *Alas for those that never sing,*
> *But die with all their music in them!*

For almost twenty-five years she lived as a recluse in her
father's house and was regarded as a "half-cracked spinster"
(Higginson's phrase). Her neatly wrapped bundles of verse were
opened only after her death. She left seclusion only to be treated
for ill-described eye trouble in Boston, suffered from spells of
"transport," "buzzing in the brain," and vertigo as "a Plank in
Reason broke." She shunned company and the light, dressed in
long-sleeved, high-collared white dresses, and eventually died of
what appeared to have been puffy-eyed renal disease. One wonders what the results would have been of a specific test for antibodies to nucleic acids. Her tale leaves the spoor of systemic

lupus erythematosus, that sad disease of young women which also singes the brain. But does the diagnosis of her malady—whatever it was—matter?

Biography can describe, but not explain, the poet. The myth of the mad poet antedates the Greeks, and, sure enough, diseases of body or spirit seem to squeeze poetry out of *some* poets. Still, not every nephritic spinster in Massachusetts or luetic *hachisch-iste* in Paris has written immortal verse. And not every neurasthenic with a famous family has kept a journal as breathtaking as Alice James's—the Darwin women might serve as age- and rank-matched controls. The lesson from literary experiments as successful as those of Dickinson and James is that the human nature they explore is not only their own. The rest of us, the poetically challenged, may not be able to play the music of despair, but we have heard its dismal tune. The madness or the music, or both, reach out from poems such as theirs to grab us and make us listen to one voice and one voice only, carefully. That experience is not unlike the clinical encounter every doctor has had, that moment when "the longing, pallid victim stretches out a sickly tendril"—perhaps even to hand us two daylilies—and says, "Listen, I have something to tell you . . ."

Nowadays we no longer believe that mental disease, be it due to familial depression, lupus erythematosus, or schizophrenia, constitutes for anyone what Henry said of Alice James: "the only solution for her of the practical problem of life." Most of us believe that the day is not far off when we will identify those inborn errors of genetic metabolism we now recognize as one form of mental illness or other. The silly days of R. D. Laing and Jacques Lacan are behind us when even schizophrenia was to be understood as "a special strategy that the patient invents in order to live an unlivable situation." The lives of our modern poets—Robert Lowell, John Berryman, Sylvia Plath, Elizabeth Bishop, for starters—show us that mental pain and self-destruction can be turned into compelling art. But until the biological roots of these symptoms are discovered, we will not be able to decide whether poetry per se is contingent on madness. It seems likely that when the genes of depression and schizophrenia are straightened out, the balance in numbers will not change between madmen and poets. Meanwhile, the afflicted are more in need of interest, attention—and asylum—than of praise. When Foucault's introduction to his English readers argues that "madness has in our age become some sort of lost truth," one wonders whether that truth is worth all those unhappy years of pain, paralysis, and solitude. Alice James, who spent her life waiting for the pain to stop, would have spotted the cant in Foucault.

Before medicine became, in Lewis Thomas's words, the Youngest Science, it was, in the words of Hippocrates, the Oldest Art. Our new science doesn't threaten the art, but perhaps the pseudoscience of our insolent machines and rattletrap gadgets is making medical care so complicated that there may be no art left. The voices of patients far humbler than Alice James or Emily Dickinson remind us that what doctors do for a living is still properly referred to as an art: as in "Life is short, but the Art long." And although doctors have entered the age of molecular medicine, have caught up with Emerson and have "taken protoplasm and mixed hydrogen, oxygen and carbon and made an animalcule"—those elements to which we have been reduced seem to be—well—so barren. Biology may be the science of life, but it becomes succulent only when it is tempered by art. George Eliot spelled this out in a letter of 1869 which remains a fine caution in the epoch of genes:

> The consideration of molecular physics is not the direct ground of human love and moral action, any more than it is the direct means of composing a noble picture or of enjoying great music. One might as well hope to dissect one's own body and be merry in doing it, as take molecular physics (in

which you must banish from your field of view what is specifically human) to be your dominant guide, your determinant of motives, in what is solely human. That every study has its bearing on every other is true; but pain and relief, love and sorrow, have their peculiar history which makes an experience and knowledge over and above the swing of atoms.

12. DR. DOYLE AND THE
CASE OF THE GUILTY GENE

Edgar Allan Poe may have written the first mystery, but Dr.
Arthur Conan Doyle put the genre on the map for keeps.
Those ever-popular stories written by Doyle and Poe share a
genre: the hero is an omniscient, eccentric detective; the narrator
is his obtuse roommate; the police are severely befuddled; the
solution hinges on recourse to natural history or the pharma-
copoeia. Most of all they celebrate what Poe has called "the
mental features discoursed of as the analytical." However, despite the similiarities in their fiction, Poe and Doyle were very
unlike with respect to fortune, temperament, and career. They
differed as much from each other as, let us say, doctor and patient. Doyle went as a medic to war against the Boers, while
"poor Edgar" died of drink and tuberculosis in the hospital.
They're also as different as checkers and chess.

The Murders in the Rue Morgue begins with a curious introduction, a mini-essay in which Poe contrasts the "analytic powers" needed for chess and checkers. He argues that the mental
features required in "the elaborate frivolity of chess" rank on a
lower scale than those wanted to solve the "unostentatious"
game of draughts (checkers). In chess, he claims, "the attention
is here called powerfully into play . . . it is the more concentra-
tive rather than the more acute player who conquers," whereas
in the simpler game of checkers, "what advantages are obtained
by either party are obtained by superior *acumen* . . . by some
recherché movement." Reading Poe's argument in the context

of his squabble with the Harvard professors, we have a hint of what he was up to when he proposed:

> Between ingenuity and the analytic ability there exists a difference far greater indeed than between the fancy and the imagination but of a character very strictly analogous. It will be found, in fact, that the ingenious are always fanciful, and the truly imaginative never otherwise than analytic.

Since Poe accused the Boston literati, and especially the Transcendentalists, of excess fancy and limited imaginations, we might read his homage to the "truly imaginative" as an advertisement for himself. Poe, champion of the recherché in his tales of terror and the imagination, seems to anticipate how critics of the future might distinguish his work from that of his disciple, Sir Arthur Conan Doyle. It's the difference between England and France, chess and checkers. The good doctor's very Anglo-Saxon hero, Sherlock Holmes, excels in the attentive power of a chess player. On the other hand, Poe's Auguste Dupin shows the acumen of a Gallic champion at draughts with his recherché move into Cuvier. "King me!" the story seems to be saying: "The ape did it!"

Poe's quest for Whodunit, in which the murderer ranks among the highest of apes, suggests that the detective story had other overtones from its beginning. *The Murders in the Rue Morgue* were committed in those critical years for natural history between the theories of Lamarck (1809) and those of Charles Darwin (1859). Baron Cuvier's original encyclopedia of the animal kingdom showed European man standing first in the Great Chain of Being, followed closely by the great apes. As one might expect, a very Gallic man was depicted at the head of the human pack, with the other specimens (Asian, Semitic, African) trailing backward to the beasts. The apes were described as "almost human, but with distinctly violent and bestial features."

With Cuvier as a template, it may not be too fanciful to suggest that the murder mystery began as a search for the ape beneath the skin, the *biology* of social guilt. And so, notwithstanding the differences between attention and acumen, checkers and chess, that Poe used to explain why he invented the genre, one has a hunch that the detective story is out not only to find Whodunit but also to search for the guilty gene.

Slightly more than a century ago, in December 1892, there appeared in *The Bookman* a review of Dr. Arthur Conan Doyle's recently published *The Adventures of Sherlock Holmes*. The piece was written by Dr. Joseph Bell, a professor of surgery at the University of Edinburgh. Since readers of that popular literary magazine knew that the Scottish surgeon was the real-life prototype of Dr. Doyle's detective—Doyle had been Bell's student and assistant—they believed that they were reading a review of Sherlock Holmes's adventures written by Sherlock Holmes himself. Bell wrote:

The greatest stride that has been made of late years in preventive and diagnostic medicine is the recognition and differentiation by bacteriological research of those minute organisms which disseminate cholera and fever, tubercle and anthrax. The importance of the infinitely little is incalculable. Poison a well at Mecca with the cholera bacillus, and the holy water which the pilgrims carry off in their bottles will infect a continent, and the rags of the victims of the plague will terrify every seaport in Christendom. Trained as he has been to appreciate minute detail, Dr. Doyle saw how he could interest his intelligent readers by taking them into his confidence, and showing his mode of working. He created a shrewd, quick-sighted, inquisitive man, half doctor, half virtuoso, with plenty of spare time, a retentive memory for whom the petty results of environment, the sign-manuals of labour, the stains of trade, the incidents of travel, have living interest, as they tend to satisfy an insatiable, almost inhuman, because impersonal curiosity.

Dr. Bell might have been describing himself. But Bell was not the only model for Dr. Doyle's half doctor, half virtuoso. And although the records are murky, it should come as no surprise that Sherlock Holmes owes as much to the Autocrat of the Breakfast Table as to the admirable Dr. Bell. Doyle has made it clear in his memoirs that he borrowed "Dr. Watson" from the surname of a fellow practitioner in Portsmouth, a Dr. James Watson. But extensive searches of Doyle's memoirs, correspondence, and scrapbooks have yielded not a word as to the origin of the name Holmes. Is there a secret? And if so, what does the secret tell us about Sir Arthur Conan Doyle and his search for the genetically guilty?

Dr. Bell tells us that a medical diagnostician and a detective share an imagination "capable of weaving a theory or piecing together a broken chain or unraveling a tangled clue." Well, it may be almost elementary—so to speak—to piece together a chain of evidence that traces the invention of Sherlock Holmes to the best-known doctor-writer of the nineteenth century: Dr. Holmes, the *Autocrat*, *Poet*, and *Professor at the Breakfast Table*, to name but three of his volumes. Indeed, I would argue that the young Dr. Doyle not only appropriated Holmes's last name for his hero but also followed the Autocrat's path to literary fame by playing the patriot card. Unfortunately, he also carried the biological Darwinism of Holmes to its social extreme. Conan Doyle got into the business of looking for guilty genes early in his career.

In September 1892, when young Dr. Doyle was by no means a household name, it was announced in the press that the *Foudroyant*, Admiral Nelson's old flagship, had been sold to the Germans—and for scrap, at that. Doyle boiled over and dispatched these verses to the press as "A Humble Petition":

> *Who says the Nation's purse is lean,*
> *Who fears for claim or bond or debt*

When all the glories that have been
Are scheduled as a cash asset?

If times are black and trade is slack,
If coal and cotton fail at last,
We've something left to barter yet—
Our glorious past . . .

There's many a crypt in which lies hid
The dust of statesman or of king;
There's Shakespeare's home to raise a bid,
And Milton's house its price would bring.

What for the sword that Cromwell drew?
What for Prince Edward's coat of mail?
What for our Saxon Alfred's tomb?
They're all for sale!

What was it that prompted this outburst of poetry in a newspaper, by a writer known to Dr. Bell and readers of *The Bookman* as "a born story teller" who wrote for magazines? It seems likely that the example, in both sentiment and meter, was that of Oliver Wendell Holmes. In September 1830, there had appeared a short notice in *The Boston Daily Advertiser* that the frigate *Constitution*, proud veteran of the American Navy, was about to be dismantled. Young Holmes—not yet a medical student, but already the class poet of Harvard '29—dashed off a poem to *The Advertiser*. That poem, "Old Ironsides," like Doyle's plea for the *Foudroyant*, was an indignant response to a tightwad regime. It gained for Holmes an immediate national reputation. Indeed, until television stamped out juvenile literacy on this continent, generations of American schoolchildren knew Holmes's poem by heart:

Ay tear her tattered ensign down!
Long has it waved on high,

And many an eye has danced to see
  That banner in the sky;
Beneath it rang the battle shout,
  And burst the cannon's roar;—
The meteor of the ocean air
  Shall sweep the clouds no more.

Her deck, once red with heroes' blood,
  Where knelt the vanquished foe,
When winds were hurrying o'er the flood,
  And waves were white below,
No more shall feel the victor's tread,
  Or know the conquered knee;—
The harpies of the shore shall pluck
  The eagle of the sea!

The poem was so well known in America that several generations of medical students used to recite a parody that began "Ay tear her tattered enzyme down . . ."

Ample evidence suggests that Doyle was a close reader of American writers: the late John Dickson Carr was not the only critic to note the strong influence of Bret Harte on the doctor's earliest adventure stories (e.g., *The American's Tale*, 1879), and Edgar Allan Poe's *Murders in the Rue Morgue* became his immediate example. Dr. Doyle's notebooks and the drafts for *A Study in Scarlet* clearly show that he turned his attention to a procedural puzzle after abandoning a murder tale inspired by Poe. In keeping with his Gallic model, Doyle was going to call it *The Lerouge Case*; you'll recall that the hero of Poe's "The Gold Bug" is named Le Grand. But rouge turned scarlet, and Doyle's notebooks show him groping for a method: "The coat-sleeve, the trouser-knee, the callosities of the forefinger and thumb, the boot—any one of these might tell us, but that all united should fail to enlighten the trained observation is incredible."

Doyle knew that in order to turn clinical observation into a story he required not only a new method but also a new kind of character who might apply that method. He needed an observer, an experimentalist who would make criminal investigation an exact science. "By a study of minutiae, footprints, mud, dust, the use of chemistry and anatomy and geology, he must reconstruct the scene of a murder as though he had been there."

While Joseph Bell was a good enough model for a detective who could *observe* the minutiae of evidence, clinical observation was only one talent required of a "stoop-shouldered wizard of lens and microscope." No; Doyle needed someone of more quantitative bent, someone who might be scholar enough to write a monograph describing "one hundred and fourteen varieties of tobacco ash." For that model Doyle required a specialist: an anatomist, a microscopist, a physiologist. And who was more qualified to serve as that model than the Parkman Professor of Anatomy and Physiology of Harvard, the doctor-poet who had introduced histology to America, Dr. Oliver Wendell Holmes? Moreover, there is little doubt that Dr. Holmes must have been very much on Dr. Doyle's mind in March and April 1886.

Sherlock Holmes makes his first appearance from behind a chemistry bench in St. Bartholomew's Hospital, where Dr. Watson mistakes him for a medical student—Holmes is working on a test for occult blood that will replace the time-tested guaiac method. The book in which the detective first appears is *A Study in Scarlet*, written in the spring of 1886. And in the spring of 1886 the life and times of one doctor were being celebrated in every British newspaper. Oliver Wendell Holmes ranked at the time with Emerson, Lowell, Longfellow, and Hawthorne in British esteem. He had arrived on a triumphant hundred-day tour of England, in the course of which he received honorary degrees from Oxford, Cambridge, and—oh yes—Edinburgh. The doctor's doings on the London social scene were duly recorded; there were literary dinners with Robert Browning, Henry James, Walter Pater, and George du Maurier; state re-

ceptions with a brace of dukes and earls at the side of the Prime
Minister (Gladstone); visits to the poet laureate (Tennyson) and
to the Derby (with Prince Albert Edward); professional recep-
tions where his companions were Sir James Paget (of the disease)
and Sir William Gull (of the thyroid). Such were the joys—
young Dr. Conan Doyle must have noticed—of a successful
career in literature and medical science.

Added to this celebrity was Holmes's association with one of
the most notorious criminal trials of the century. Every English connoisseur of murder was aware of the Webster-Parkman
case, the Harvard Medical School murder of 1849. As Simon
Schama has reminded us in *Dead Certainties*, John Webster, the
Erving Professor of Chemistry, was accused of having killed,
dismembered, and almost destroyed the remains of Dr. George
Parkman. Dr. Parkman, a wealthy practitioner and sharp busi-
nessman, had given the land on which the Harvard Medical
School stood, and the university rewarded him by naming the
chair of anatomy and physiology after him. Dean Holmes, who
occupied that chair, testified for the prosecution. As an expert
witness he had confirmed that "a large mass of human bones,
fused slag and cinders . . . the block of mineral teeth and the
gold filling" found in the ovens of Professor Webster's chemistry laboratory were the remains of the unfortunate Parkman.
These residues were also identified by Holmes's anatomical colleague Dr. Wyman—he of the Philosopher's Camp in the Adirondacks. Their careful analyses helped the prosecution to
prove foul play and to uncover Dr. Webster's postmortem high
jinks with the body. (One might say he was the first Harvard
biochemist found guilty of cooking the data.) Detailed accounts
of the trial in the English press never failed to mention Dr.
Holmes. A few years after Webster was convicted and hanged,
Charles Dickens, one of many English fans of that grisly crime,
persuaded Dr. Holmes to walk him through Harvard's chemistry lab to view Webster's furnace, proof that every English

literary gent knew that the Parkman professor was privy to the secrets of the Parkman case.

We have ample reason, therefore, for supposing that Doyle conflated several aspects of Dr. Holmes in his detective hero. The name, certainly. The doctor-author model, probably. The forensic bent, surely. But the scientific urges? That numerical drive? Do these derive from Bell the surgeon or Holmes the physician? Holmes, on the evidence, one might argue. Holmes, as we've seen, had been trained in the quantitative school of Louis and drilled in that motto *Formez toujours les idées nettes* . . . Dr. Holmes paraphrased it as: "Always make sure that you form a distinct and clear idea of the matter you are considering. Always avoid vague approximations where exact estimates are possible; *about so many—about so much*—instead of the precise number and quantity." Those words might have dropped from the mouth of Sherlock Holmes when Watson lowered his newspaper, as he did in *The Resident Patient*, to look up at an unframed picture on the wall of Henry Ward Beecher (brother of Harriet Beecher Stowe, lifelong friend and correspondent of Dr. Holmes). They do, in fact, practically drop from the mouth of Dr. Stamford in *A Study in Scarlet* as he describes Holmes to Watson: "He appears to have a passion for exact and definite knowledge." *Fuyez toujours le à peu près,* Stamford might have said.

Holmes returned from his studies in France fully aware of his responsibility for introducing new methods into a medical backwater: "I have lived among a great, a glorious people; I have thrown my thoughts into a new language; I have received the shock of new minds and new habits." Once at Harvard, he inaugurated the study of medical microscopy in the United States. He went on to design a number of teaching and research microscopes, inventing a portable microscope for use in the classroom. Following the lead of Samuel F. B. Morse, who had brought the daguerreotype back from *his* Paris sojourn, Holmes became an ardent photographer. The best-known portraits of Dr. Holmes depict him in his study, posed in front of a microscope or the odd optical instrument. He was most proud of his achievements in histology, of what the achromatic lens had wrought, asking his Harvard students in 1861:

> Now what have we come to in our own day? In the first place, the minute structure of all the organs has been made out in the most satisfactory way. The special arrangements of the vessels and the ducts of all the glands, of the air-tubes and vesicles of the lungs, of the parts which make up the skin and other membranes, all the details of those complex parenchymatous organs which had confounded investigation so long, have been lifted out of the invisible into the sight of all observers . . . Everywhere we find cells, modified or unchanged. They roll in inconceivable multitudes (5 million or more to the cubic milliliter) as blood whisks through our vessels . . . they preside over the chemical processes which elaborate the living fluids [and] the soul itself sits on a throne of nucleated cells.

Professor Holmes throbbed with satisfaction at the new world under his lens. He did not foresee that, in less than a generation, the routine use of portable and powerful microscopes in the field would turn the sanitary revolution into the bacteriological revolution. He *did* anticipate Dr. Bell's tribute to the importance of the infinitely little. Indeed, the passage leads us to suspect that a lean sleuth with lens and microscope was exactly what a young medical writer *would* come up with who had been weaned on the teachings of Bell and the writings of Holmes. For Holmes was more than a sedentary professor of anatomy. As a physiologist he had moved to more kinetic studies. He had written scholarly and popular articles on the gait of man and beast: footprints on the sands of time. Lens in hand, he pointed out to his Harvard classes that anatomy studies the organism in space whereas physiology studies it in time. And when Sidney Paget went on to draw the restless Sherlock Holmes, it was also before a microscope or with lens in hand. There, fixed on the pages of childhood the lean sleuth will forever peer through the lens at the spoor in the mud: "Quick, Watson, the game's afoot!" Dr. Doyle took from Dr. Holmes's thirteen volumes of writing the lesson that experimental science could produce a popular literature. Private investigation could bring popular fame. "And is it no accident," to ask Holmes's question again, that by the end of the nineteenth century, doctors who studied disease began to call themselves clinical *investigators* rather than clinical *observers*? Sure enough, by the time the American Society for Clinical Investigation was founded at the turn of the century, both doctor and detective had become investigators; both used the microscope to study the importance of the infinitely little.

✳

The shift from observation to investigation also took place in the nineteenth-century novel. The literary scholar Lawrence Rothfield has observed in *Vital Signs* (1992) that the displacement of realism (Balzac) by naturalism (Zola) correlated in time and sensibility with the "displacement of one form of scientific thought (that of clinical medicine) by another (that of experimental medicine)." What Rothfield has called the "invasive aspects" of clinical and criminal investigation led him to explore the Freudian roots of detective fiction. He suggested that the pleasures of criminal investigation are almost erotic. Holmes sloshes through bog and moor to glimpse—at last—the primal scene. The detective, with nostrils dilated, cheeks flushed, hot after the scent of a criminal—or the literal denouement of the family romance—resembles in his rush of excitement the scientist who has snared an offending microbe: "Yes, I have found it!"

But Poe was always ahead of Doyle, even in the Freudian

sweepstakes. Here is his portrait of the Chevalier Auguste Dupin in deductive rapture at the moment of discovery: "His manner at these moments was frigid and abstract; his eyes were vacant in expression; while his voice, usually a rich tenor, rose to a treble . . ." Poe precedes this orgasmic description with another that tells us as much about Watson and Holmes as about the narrator and Dupin: "He boasted to me . . . that most men, in respect to himself, wore windows in their bosoms, and was wont to follow up such assertions by direct and very startling proofs of his intimate knowledge of my own." Oliver Wendell Holmes wrote what he called his medicated novels to provide popular, sensational entertainment, and Rothfield could have had Holmes of Boston, rather than Conan Doyle of Edinburgh, in mind when he describes the "sensational effects that detection can produce in the detected, the detective and the reader—effects that themselves are being given a scientific, even medical, status at the very moment when the detective story comes into its own as a genre: the moment of Holmes." But the moment of Holmes—which was also the moment of naturalism—had Darwinian as well as Freudian undertones. Doctor and detective alike used the tools of science to root out the abnormal in body or body politic. It is probably again no accident that Francis Galton (1822–1911), who founded the science of eugenics, developed fingerprinting by microscopy as part of his campaign of racial classification (1891). And eugenics turned out to be the applied science of social Darwinism. As Dr. Bell pointed out: "Racial peculiarities, hereditary tricks of manner, accent, occupation or the want of it, education, environment of all kinds, by their little trivial impressions gradually mould or carve the individual, and leave finger marks or chisel sores which the expert can recognize."

Here then was a new scientific method to find the ape beneath the skin, to search in the odd thumbprint for those racial peculiarities which only the expert can recognize! Galton himself makes an appearance in the penultimate paragraph of Dr. Bell's review. Galton's fingerprint method, Bell argued, renders "the ridges and furrows of the stain visible and permanent." Those stains were racial and indelible. No wonder that we nowadays call the technique used to identify DNA fragments by restriction enzymes (RFLP) "fingerprinting."

Informed by hindsight, we can accuse a literature based on Galtonian eugenics of social Darwinism. In *The Adventures of Sherlock Holmes* and its sequels, moral flaws are signified by physical abnormalities. Doyle offers us stock villains aplenty: the Gipsy, the Moor, the Levantine, the Man with the Blue Carbuncle. Those *others.* The detective ferrets out their guilt not from behavior alone but from Bell's "myriads of signs eloquent and instructive which need the educated eye to detect." Each twist of the spine, droop of a lid, bend in the nose, or blotch on the skin is an outward sign of a deeper flaw in the flesh. Those racial stains, which offend the physical standards of a settled race, are as visible and permanent as a fingerprint. The genes they express are the genes of guilt. Sherlock Holmes presided over the most thrilling gene hunt of his century and became a hero of adolescents worldwide. Meanwhile, Sir Arthur Conan Doyle became the staunch dean of Empire loyalists and—like Yeats and William James before him—lapsed into spiritualism in old age. But as a student of Dr. Bell and fan of Dr. Holmes, Dr. Doyle put on the map forever the notion that doctors and detectives are after the same game: "Quick, Watson, the game's afoot!" It was the moment of Holmes indeed.

After the moment of Holmes, in fact as in fiction, it became the task of clinical and criminal investigators—of docs and cops—to root out the transgressor, to incriminate man or microbe. Edmund Wilson described what happens to a villain in the nineteenth-century detective story: "He has been caught by an infallible power, the supercilious and omniscient detective, who knows exactly where to fix the guilt." We have learned

over the last century that social Darwinists—detective or
dictator—have had no qualms about fixing guilt on one or another gene. If this lesson smacks of anachronism, so be it.

The rise of the detective story in the years between Lamarck
and Darwin is one aspect of the nineteenth-century argument in
favor of nature over nurture. In that sense, murder is no mystery; when a detective scans the palm or the face he is reading
the gene. Holmes's Elsie Venner, Doyle's Moriarty, even Poe's
ourang-outang are cast as losers in the Darwinian lottery, examples of *others* who could no more change their nature than
their serpentine eye or their furrow of skin. On the other hand,
a meliorist would argue that if guilt lies in the gene, the guilty
are more to be pitied than censured. That is exactly what Oliver
Wendell Holmes *did* argue in *Elsie Venner*. Those whom Dr.
Doyle and the social Darwinists turned into villains, Dr. Holmes
and the Boston meliorists regarded as victims. Snakebit in the
womb but guiltless before God, they were more to be pitied
than censured. What is given by nature can be forgiven by man.
Following that example today, we might say that if "special influences" work on behavior like ferments in the blood, it is the
task of our new genetics to give them any other name but guilt.

Dr. Doyle may not have learned genetic sweetness and light
from Dr. Holmes, but he remained forever in the Autocrat's
debt for the name of his sleuth. On his first trip to America in
the autumn of 1894, he visited Boston to view Mount Auburn
Cemetery. Among the russet elms, yellow willows, and golden
maples, he saw the graves of those who had presided over the
Flowering of New England: "Lowell, Longfellow, Channing,
Brooks, Agassiz, Parkman and very many more." But he did
one other thing. "Yesterday," he wrote, "I visited Oliver Wendell Holmes' grave and I laid a big wreath on it." Why Holmes
of all the others? Elementary, my dear Watson!

13. THE BACTERIOLOGICAL
REVOLUTION

The standard of medical instruction [in Paris], the facility with which all is obtained, and the rapidity with which instruction is acquired, convince me that the attentive student may return a sounder physician at twenty-five than many who slumber till sixty in our own languid scientific atmosphere. The truth is, I live at Paris just as if I had been there all my life, and indeed I can hardly conceive of anybody's living in any other way, so completely have I naturalized myself. It seems hideous to think of more than two meals a day; how could I ever have dined at two o'clock? How could I have put anything to my mouth but a silver fork? How could I have survived dinner without a napkin? . . . Give my love to everybody.

—Oliver Wendell Holmes, letter to his parents, June 1831

Oliver Wendell Holmes and Elizabeth Blackwell went to France to learn medicine and, like most students in Paris, learned as much from the city as from books. The Paris to which these young provincials came was the intellectual center of the West, but it was also the center of recurrent revolutions—and of cholera. Holmes arrived on the rue Monsieur-le-Prince in 1830 after the July Revolution had put Louis Philippe on the throne, and Elizabeth Blackwell arrived at the Maternité after the king's overthrow in 1848. Both of those years were cholera years in Paris and throughout the world; both were years of revolution. On June 15, 1849, Blackwell wrote:

The Louvre and the Tuileries opposite were closed and filled with soldiers . . . On the bridges, at the corners of the streets, were large groups of blouses [workmen], students, citizens, women, listening to some orator of the moment, gesticulating violently. More than once I observed a woman enthusiastically haranguing an audience. The most curious mixture of passions was visible on the faces—fear, anger, indignation, hope, hatred; there was many a figure that realized the horrors of an earlier revolution.

Nowadays, social and medical historians make much of the concordance between the waves of cholera and of social unrest that swept across Europe. They tend to agree that the relationship was reciprocal: social upheaval permitted spread of disease while the threat of disease caused social upheaval. In most of Europe the epidemics took a major toll of the masses and were severe enough to frighten the classes. That same June, Alexis de Tocqueville, Minister of Foreign Affairs for the government that replaced Lamartine's, first noted the synergy between revolution and cholera:

. . . at the moment no revolution by force of arms was to be feared: but there was reason to fear a struggle; and civil war, always a cruel thing to anticipate, is much worse combined with the horrors of the plague. For cholera was ravaging Paris. On that occasion death struck all classes of society. A good many members of the Constituent Assembly had already succumbed, and Bugeaud [a general], whom Africa had spared, was dead.

The first law of social thermodynamics states that every public action breeds its own and equal reaction. One should not be surprised, therefore, that each of the cholera epidemics of 1830–32, 1848–49, and 1870–71 not only coincided with revolution but set the stage for a sharp return to order. Lethal cholera began in "septic Asia"—Auden's phrase—and the fears it aroused put police in the streets.

Cholera has always been endemic on the Indian subcontinent and remains so today, despite—one is tempted to add—centuries of alternative medicine. It was not until 1817, however, that "Asiatic cholera" found a European host. In the course of subduing the Mahratta Brahmin of southwestern India, Lord Hastings lost a third of his 10,000 British troops to the disease; the first medical reports of Asiatic cholera date no earlier than 1819. Over the next decade, the disease spread slowly from the East to the Middle East and then—via the Caucasus and Crimea—to St. Petersburg and Warsaw. Epidemic cholera finally broke out in Paris during the July Revolution of 1830. It has been argued that the angry conflicts between Turk and Greek, Pole and Russian—the wars of Byron, Lafayette, and Samuel Gridley Howe—helped to spread the disease from east to west. Tradesmen, soldiers, and refugees were the human vectors; thousands of the displaced spilled over the borders of Europe looking for shelter from Eastern despots. The Paris of the 1830s was one such refuge, and young Holmes was vastly impressed as he compared the City of Light to small-town Boston:

> One of the greatest pleasures of living abroad is to meet in such an easy, pleasant sort of a way people from all quarters of the world. Greek and Barbarian, Jew and Gentile, differ much less than one thinks at first, and this you never learn from books—or never believe. They know it well here, and you may see what we should call nigger people—that is, young black Egyptian students, of a shade between ink and charcoal, arm in arm with God's image cut in ivory.

Sure enough, those less tolerant than Holmes blamed strangers for the spread of this most foul disease: the "Gyppo," the Pole, the Greek, and the Jew. Richard J. Evans has pointed out in *Cholera in the 19th Century* that cholera presented a unique challenge to the social fabric of the West from the "uncivilized East." Cholera produces a violent, wrenching diarrhea, which within hours racks and desiccates its victims as it fouls the sickroom. It therefore challenged common assumptions of European cultural, hygienic, and biological superiority. It demonstrated the "vulnerability of even the most civilized people to a disease associated mainly with oriental backwardness." In the course of the nineteenth century, six bouts of Asian cholera struck the capital cities of the West. Oliver Wendell Holmes came to Paris at the end of the second, Blackwell and Tocqueville survived the third. In Blackwell's day as in Holmes's, all that was known about cholera was that the disease spread rapidly, its victims suffered terribly, and its mortality was as high as 50 percent.

Nowadays, we know almost everything there is to know about cholera except how to prevent the social pathology that is its proximate cause. We understand that the disease is spread when the stool of infected individuals contaminates the water supply. We have learned that the microbe multiplies in the gut and produces a toxin which when isolated can produce each of the features of the illness. We can point to the amino acid of the regulatory protein (called Ga_s) that is modified (ADP-ribosylated) by the toxin's own A subunit. We know that the Ga_s subunit activates another enzyme (adenylate cyclase). We have worked out that when this enzyme is "on" it causes the victim's intestines to pump out more salt and water through microscopic channels than if the sluices of hell were open. Moreover, if we have the remedies at hand—salt and water given by mouth or by vein—we can stop the disease in its tracks. In the end, a clean water supply and antibiotics will regularly bring things under control. The recent epidemic of cholera in Rwanda demonstrated how well we understand the physiology of the gut and how poorly the physiology of hate.

✳

That divergence between physiology and morality in our century leads us to the story of Robert Koch, a doctor who might be called the Lydgate of Wollstein, a small-town practitioner who became perhaps the greatest of microbe hunters. Plunked down in a tiny eastern German town, removed from the centers of learning, Koch set up a small laboratory in the examination room of his medical office and determined to find the cause of anthrax, which was endemic in the area. He had become interested in this disease of cattle and farmers because its lesions so clearly resulted from contact with something *infectious*. Working odd hours, scraping samples from the soil and the coarse garments of his rustic patients, he showed for the first time that a specific microbe caused a specific human disease. "Never, surely, could a man have found himself in a position less favorable for scientific research and away from the scientific appliances which are the necessary tools of the investigator," said Dr. Arthur Conan Doyle in appreciation. In the course of his work, Koch managed to discover general methods for the cultivation of microbes in the dish and to take the first photomicrographs of an infective agent, investigations that had the most far-reaching consequences. George Eliot, in 1872, might have been describing Koch when she describes Lydgate's plans in *Middlemarch*:

> There was fascination in the hope that the two purposes would illuminate each other: the careful observation and inference which was his daily work, the use of the microscopic lens to further his judgment in special cases, would further his thought as an instrument of larger inquiry. Was this not the typical pre-eminence of his profession? He would be a good Middlemarch doctor and by that very means keep himself in the track of far-reaching investigation.

Robert Koch kept himself in the track and fulfilled his motto of *nunquam otiosus*—never idle—on Christmas Day of 1875. Undisturbed by his daily round of patients, he had time to examine dishes filled with culture medium and various scrapings that he had made from infected material and maintained overnight at 37° C. The next day he noted discrete new growth in serial dilutions of the medium. He noted with proper pride that he had finally succeeded in growing a pure isolate of the bacillus that caused anthrax. He then went on to use these pure cultures to transmit the disease to experimental animals and to find the infective microbe in their lesions. Altogether, Koch spent eight years as a country doctor in Wollstein before he emerged to become world-famous for his next discovery: the tubercle bacillus. Like the fictional young Lydgate, he was hardworking, driven, and equally dedicated to patients and to the study of microbes. Unlike Lydgate, he had a disinterest in furniture and was helped by a wife who was no Rosamond Vincy. Emmy Koch described those days: "Through careful savings of money, a better microscope was obtained. How happy Robert was! There came another day of celebration when a better microtome was purchased . . . It was my job to find out first how sick a patient really was, and to send away those who didn't really need medical attention. In that way, Robert could often remain for hours at his work."

We now know that Robert's work was the beginning of the bacteriological revolution. This major assault by the countries of the West on microbial disease resulted in our understanding of the causes of infections rather than their prevention, which had been the aim of the sanitary revolution. It took almost sixty years before this effort was rewarded by the discovery of antibiotics. Nevertheless, the bacteriological revolution established the science of microbiology, a science that doubled our life span and launched the biological revolution, the Flowering of DNA. As Carl Schorske has taught us, intellectual conquest and social good were as much the aims of German social democracy as of meliorism in England and France. Good chunks of the Erfurt Manifesto (1891), the program of German social democracy, could have been written by George Eliot or George

Bernard Shaw and signed by Lloyd George, or, for that matter, by Dr. Georges Clemenceau. And although much of microbial research before the first Sarajevo was fueled by chauvinist vanity, by and large the fellowship of medical science prevailed over national pride. The legend of Robert Koch and cholera speaks of that international fellowship.

> Up to now twenty-two cholera victims and seventeen cholera patients have been examined in Calcutta, with the help of both the microscope and gelatin cultures. In all cases, the comma bacillus has been found. These results, taken together with those obtained in Egypt, prove that we have found the pathogen responsible for cholera.

So wrote Koch on February 4, 1884, from India, reporting on the success of the German Cholera Commission to his supervisors in Berlin. In July 1883, cholera had entered Egypt from India and the Arabian peninsula along the recently opened Suez Canal. Quarantine facilities were set up at major ports and at way stations for pilgrims returning from Mecca, to which Muslims from India had brought the disease. The caliphate appealed to Europe for help, rightly supposing that the century-long rivalry in science between France and Germany would prompt both countries to send the best and brightest of their new microbe hunters. Altruism was only one motive; if the disease could be halted in Egypt before it spread to the West, the fifth pandemic of Asiatic cholera might be prevented. By mid-August 1884 the two contending teams of French and German scientists were on site in Alexandria seeking to be first to isolate the cholera agent. National honor and human lives were both at stake, perhaps in that order of priority for some. The French team, which was handpicked by Pasteur himself, consisted of the internist Isador Straus, the veterinarian Edmond Nocard, and two of Pasteur's most valued assistants, Emile Roux and Louis Thuillier. Together with several Italian colleagues, they were quartered at the Hôpital Européen. The Germans were led by Koch, fresh from his triumphant discovery of the tubercle bacillus. He was assisted by the chemist Ludwig Treskow and the bacteriologists Georg Gaffky and Bernhard Fischer; they were housed in the Greek Hospital across town from the French team. (These days, doctors remember Roux, Gaffky, and Nocard as names of bacteria studied in first-year microbiology. Their fame is shared by a dirty village stopover for pilgrims on the Suez Canal; El Tor is now simply the technical name for a bad strain of the cholera vibrio.)

The French struck pay dirt soon after arrival. They found strange new microscopic structures in stained blood smears of patients with cholera. Excitement mounted, and news of the possible identification of the cholera agent spread around town. But before their preliminary finding could be confirmed, tragedy struck the French camp. Thuillier, at the age of twenty-seven the youngest of the team, succumbed within thirty-six hours to an explosive bout of cholera. As Roux reported to *Le Temps*:

> Straus and I were obliged to hold him up to prevent his fainting. From this moment everything passed involuntarily; and, in spite of the most energetic treatment, at eight o'clock he was already moribund. . . . We employed strong frictions (rubbing of the limbs). All the French and Italian doctors were present. Iced champagne and subcutaneous injections of ether were given freely. In short, everything that could be devised was done to prevent a fatal issue.

The champagne was as useless as friction and the issue *was* fatal. At Thuillier's funeral, Robert Koch and the other German scientists showed up with two wreaths for their fallen competitor. "They are only a small token, but they are of laurel and most fitting for him, who deserves such glory," said Koch, who helped to carry the coffin. Myth and legend have arisen around this episode. For it turned out that the strange new particles discovered by the French group were nothing but fractured blood *platelets* with altered staining properties. Koch is said to have realized that the French discovery must be an artifact and suspected that the real culprit was a novel microbe that resembled a punctuation mark: *"ein Komma Bazillus."* In the legend, Koch is called out in the middle of the night by a visit from the distraught Roux. The two erstwhile rivals rush through the dark, disease-ridden town to the bedside of the dying Thuillier, whom Koch has known since the young man visited him in Berlin. Thuillier looks up at the master and weakly asks his evaluation of the new "organisms" the French have spotted in the blood. "Have we found it?" asks the moribund youth. Koch wishes his colleague to die a happy man: "Yes, you have found it."

In reality—as opposed to this legend from de Kruif's *Microbe Hunters*—neither the French nor the German team made the conclusive discovery in Alexandria. Perhaps because of strict quarantine measures, perhaps because the epidemic wound down naturally with the end of hot weather, Thuillier's death was almost the last from cholera that season. The French went home with their samples and Koch proceeded to Calcutta. There the disease was still rampant, and it was in India that Koch isolated pure cultures of the cholera vibrio for the first time. He spelled out its local epidemiology and finally proved that it is spread via contaminated water. By rigorous bacteriological means, he showed that John Snow had been correct in 1854 when he concluded that water from the Broad Street pump spread the disease. In Calcutta as in London, cholera traveled in water contaminated by feces. Koch's meticulous maps of clean and contaminated water tanks in Calcutta proved to be as convincing a demonstration of how a microbe is spread as the street maps of John Snow or the maternity lists of Drs. Holmes and Semmelweis. Once the Egyptians learned that cholera was carried by pilgrims returning from Mecca, strong sanitary measures combined with enforced quarantine along the Suez Canal stopped this route from becoming a chronic portal of entry. But

the road from Mecca continued to stir the Western imagination
by combining sanitary fear with religious chauvinism. Dr. Bell,
you will recall, had also sniffed the spoor of the dirty stranger:
"The importance of the infinitely little is incalculable. Poison a
well at Mecca with the cholera bacillus, and the holy water
which the pilgrims carry off in their bottles will infect a continent, and the rags of the victims of the plague will terrify every
seaport in Christendom."

Paul de Kruif played the Oriental card in the popular prose
of his generation (1926): "It is thanks to these bold searchings
of Robert Koch that Europe and America no longer dread the
devastating raids of these puny but terrible little murderers from
the Orient—and their complete elimination from the world
waits only upon the civilization and sanitation of India." The
microbe hunters of the nineteenth century were certain that once
the causative organism of a disease was identified and its mode
of spread appreciated, sanitary measures would suffice to elim-
inate it. And if those who carried it were the immigrant, the
poor, the mad, the Gyppo, the Indian or Jew—well, so be it.
The needs of public health came first and the rights of "lesser
breeds without the law" a distant second.

✳

More than a century after Koch, no one would await expectantly
the "civilization and sanitation of India" and no public official
would link the two. We no longer believe that civilization and
sanitation go hand in hand at all, precisely because we have rejected the social Darwinism of Bell and de Kruif. We cannot
even agree on a common definition of civilization and seem—
on evidence—to have abandoned belief in the germ theory. Sad
victims of open, cavitary tuberculosis walk unfettered about the
streets of American cities, the ports of our hemisphere have become as pestilent as the El Tor of 1883, while quarantine is
reserved for rabid dogs. To use a sanitarian metaphor, we seem
to have tossed out the baby of hygiene with the bathwater of

chauvinism. In consequence, the temper of our time seems indifferent to the glory of medical discovery. In the postmodern era, we take greater interest in the fall from grace of a Jonas Salk, a Robert Gallo, or a David Baltimore than in the magic of their achievements. *Arrowsmith* and meliorism are out, the rock group Aerosmith and MTV are in.

> *I believe in rags to riches*
> *Your inheritance won't last*
> *So take your Grey Poupon my friend*
> *And shove it up your ass!*
> *CHORUS:*
> *Eat the Rich:*
> *there's only one thing that they're good for*
> *Eat the Rich:*
> *take one bite now—come back for more . . .*

The rags-to-riches rock group Aerosmith took their name from a book little read these days. Ironically, a good number of my students over the last few years have been led to read *Arrowsmith* because someone told them that the rock group was based on a "doctor book." They've found it quaint, dated, and totally inspiring. Martin Arrowsmith, in turn, was inspired by the microbe hunters, and Sinclair Lewis has Martin resolve that if he had to be "a small town doctor he would be such a small town doctor as Robert Koch." Unlike Aerosmith's grungy millionaires, Arrowsmith leaves riches not for rags but for science; his earliest ambition matches that of young Dr. Lydgate, a character who would "do good small work for Middlemarch and great work for the world." Martin Arrowsmith's picaresque career blends the biographies of Paul de Kruif and Sinclair Lewis's father: research in a bacteriology lab in Michigan, a small-town doctor's life in Wisconsin, work at the Rockefeller Institute, the temptations of money and the flesh. Eventually Martin and his wife travel to a Caribbean island to stop an outbreak of the pneumonic plague. On that plague-ridden island, Martin's Swedish colleague is killed by the epidemic they have been fighting; his death is the heroic death of Thuillier:

> "What is it? What is it?" "I t'ink—it's got me. Some flea got me. Yes," in a shaky but extremely interested manner, "I was yoost thinking I will go and quarantine myself. I have fever all right and adenitis . . . O my God, Martin, I am so weak! Not scared . . . It hurts some, but life was a good game. And—I am a pious agnostic. Oh, Martin, give my people the phage! Save all of them—"

Somewhere in the firmament of fiction the young Lydgate and Martin Arrowsmith must be chuckling over Aerosmith and Grey Poupon. Fever in the flesh has another meaning these days:

> *It's got me all soaking wet*
> *FLESH—the only thing that's worth the sweat*
> *From the Mississippi River*
> *To the highest mountain in Tibet . . .*
> *From a Sufi in a rickshaw to a bimbo in a pink Corvette*
> *Everybody gotta have*
> *FLESH!*

In our twentieth century *fin de siècle*, the Sufi and the bimbo, not to speak of Norman Mailer and Shirley MacLaine, appear convinced that the causal notions of Western medical science cannot account for the facts of human health and disease. The media fans of Eastern medicine and the millionaires of drug rock do not await de Kruif's age of civilization and sanitation; for them it is not even desirable:

> *I got a rip in my pants and a hole in my brand new shoes*
> *I got a Margarita nose and a breath full of Mad Dog Booze*
> *CHORUS:*

I got the fever, fever, fever
Yeah, we're all here cause we're not all there tonight

As we slouch to our millennium dulled by fever, fever, fever, it seems more than a short century ago that meliorist and microbe hunter marched together. But in the years before the two world wars and the two Sarajevos, men of goodwill in the lands of the West believed that the armies of health and reason wore the same uniform. Roux and Koch, Frenchman and German, marched together under the white ensign of sanitation. Under that banner, science went on to conquer anthrax and typhoid, diphtheria and plague. It had less luck with unreason. Jacques Loeb—the model for Dr. Gottlieb in *Arrowsmith*—numbered Robert Koch among the men of reason, among the *philosophes* who "dared to follow the consequences of a mechanistic science, incomplete as it then was, and apply them to the rules of human conduct, and who thereby laid the foundation of tolerance, justice and gentleness which was the hope of our civilization until it was buried under the wave of homicidal emotion which swept through the world in 1914."

It could be said that the dream of nineteenth-century reason was interrupted in 1914 by the Guns of August and became a nightmare awaiting Judgment at Nuremberg.

In January 1946, the dapper Dr. Claus Schilling appeared before the War Crimes Tribunal in Nuremberg. Schilling had retired in 1936 as director of tropical medicine at the Robert Koch Institute in Berlin, founded before World War I thanks to the generous gift of Andrew Carnegie, that Undershaft of American philanthropy. When Koch had come to America in 1908 to visit his two immigrant brothers in the Midwest, the liberal German-American Medical Association had convened a testimonial dinner in New York at which Koch thanked the sanitarians in America for their work in public hygiene. (There were at the time no prominent microbe hunters in the United States.) He was pleased that among the guests was Andrew Carnegie and he promised his benefactor that the work of the Koch Institute would "be an international affair, benefiting all mankind. And we have to thank Mr. Carnegie for placing this institution on a sound financial basis. *Herr Carnegie, lebe hoch!*"

Well, the only ones living *hoch* under Schilling had been the National Socialists. In 1941, Schilling was as happily retired in Mussolini's Italy as were George Santayana and Ezra Pound and equally satisfied with the benefits of fascism. But his former colleagues informed him of a unique opportunity to resume his work on experimental malaria. Dr. Leonardo Conti, the Reich Public Health Director (sic!), told Schilling that facilities had become available for work on malaria in humans. In the finest tradition of National Socialism, Schilling came out of retirement to fiddle with *Homo sapiens*. At Dachau, Schilling was able to infect more than a thousand inmates with *vivax* or *falciparum* malaria; scores died and of those unwilling subjects who survived, many suffered from disabling, intercurrent infections. In adjacent wards, Dr. Franz Blaha carried on experiments on the effects of sulfa drugs on wound infections. He told the tribunal about Dr. Schilling's malaria work and his own experimental protocols:

> Forty healthy men were used at a time. All treatment was forbidden for three days, by which time serious inflammation and in many cases general blood poisoning had occurred. In some cases, all the limbs were amputated. For these experiments, Polish, Czech, and Dutch priests were ordinarily used. Most of the six hundred to eight hundred persons who were used finally died. Most of the others became permanent invalids and were later killed.

Dr. Schilling of the Robert Koch Institute presented what in those days may have been a novel excuse. He was only following orders! And when an outraged American prosecutor from Newark, Major John J. Monigan, pointed out that the Nazi doctor had voluntarily left retirement to work at Dachau, Dr. Schilling pleaded that his malaria experiments were not so gruesome as those in which the Dutch priests were dismembered. "Besides," he pleaded, "my will was not to occupy myself with what did not belong to my laboratory. I did my work in the camp and didn't look right or left."

Right or left, the orders he was only following were those of his colleagues in public health. Dr. Conti and Dr. Karl Brandt, the Reich Commissioner for Health and Sanitation, had in 1940 presided over the extermination of the *Ausschusskinder* (literally, garbage children) in a crippled children's institution at Grafeneck in Württemberg. Those crippled or mentally defective children were the first of all Nazi victims to be gassed and cremated. With all the authority of the sanitary and bacteriological revolutions behind them, the Nazi doctors kept the curious away by posting over the doors of this the first of their crematoria:

ACHTUNG: EPIDEMIE!

Between the philanthropic sentiments of Roux and Koch in Alexandria and the cruel falsehoods of Conti and Schilling at Dachau lie the sorry years of fascism and the misuse of science in the twentieth century. Now that we have resumed the long, slow march of meliorist medicine, it may be useful to remember the lessons of cholera and fascism. The disease was conquered by an open, intellectual competition among scientists of many nations, each committed to the skeptical tradition of Western reason. At its best, that tradition was laced with the kindness of the Koch legend: "Yes, you have found it." On the other hand, the Nazis based their movement on a popular resentment of established political parties, appeals to national honor and "family values" fueled by an open antipathy to "cultural elites."

We are told frequently nowadays that the expensive, auto-

cratic medical science of our day has substituted its own elite
values for those that would better serve one or another of our
subcultures. It seems to me that I have heard that song before.
It's from an old familiar score. Dr. Karl Gebhardt told Major
Monigan that Hitler and his lieutenants

> were all attracted to "natural medicine" . . . they had a child-
> ish enthusiasm. All sorts of popular drugs which were not
> approved by the medical profession allegedly because we did
> not understand them or were too conceited or were finan-
> cially interested in the suppression of them, were used exper-
> imentally in concentration camps . . . What the National
> Socialists wanted to do was to introduce a popular medicine.

In the mid-1990s, cholera lurks not only in Rwanda. We are, in
fact, in the midst of the seventh worldwide pandemic of cholera.
The strains that infect the warmer regions of the earth are related
to the nasty El Tor strain. Since their appearance in Peru in 1991
the vibrios have infected over a million in the Western Hemisphere alone. Happily enough, the mortality of cholera is now
minimal, thanks to rapid intervention and public health measures. Meanwhile good vaccines based on recombinant DNA are
already in the field: a live oral vaccine in which the A subunit
gene has been deleted has proved to be about 85 percent effective. We therefore have good reason to hope that the Flowering
of DNA will end the vibrio's reign.

Nevertheless, the El Tor strain is poking across the Rio
Grande: by September 1994, a sample had been identified in the
Croton water system of New York. From ports in Costa Rica
to Haiti, cholera is knocking at our southern border. But the
vibrio is not our only recurrent pandemic. In 1995, fascism lurks
not only in Rome. Mobs again hail Mussolini in the Piazza Ve-
nezia and skinheads shout hatred from the soccer stands. The
death camps never existed says the Canadian doubter on the
tube. Swastikas decorate the helmets of Hell's Angels in Oak-

land and deface the doors of synagogues in Boston. The themes of *Blut und Boden*, nativism, National Socialism—of mindless violence—are heard from Stuttgart to Lyon, Kiev to Zagreb, Shreveport to Houston. The militias of Rush Limbaugh and the fans of Aerosmith share enemies with Drs. Schilling and Gebhardt; unreason has targets other than the Flowering of DNA.

"Such are the blows cholera can strike at the end of an epidemic!" wrote Roux to Pasteur after young Thuillier died. We will have to find a proper response to the last blows of the fascist epidemic of our century, lest—like cholera—it continues to rub against our border, itching to get in. Most likely, what worked for meliorist and microbe hunter should work again, civilization and sanitation. That response should echo those reassuring words, "Yes, you have found it."

14. DNA AND DR. HOLMES

The main value science has to offer for the practical solution of a problem is its method, which created science itself. The essential point about the scientific method is that it meets problems as problems . . . irrespective of prejudices and chauvinism. We do not ask who is right, but ask what the truth is. Searching for the truth we collect data and analyze them with cool heads, with uncompromising honesty, unbiased by interest or sentiment, fear or hatred.

—Albert Szent-Györgyi, *The Naked Ape*, 1970

It is then, very superficial to speak of science as being a common property of mankind, equally accessible to all peoples and classes and offering them all an equal field of work. The problems of science do not present themselves in the same way to all men. The Negro and the Jew will view the same world in a different way from the German investigator.

—H. Rust, Minister of Education in the Third Reich, c. 1938, quoted by W. B. Cannon, *The Way of an Investigator*, 1945

These two comments obviously express two very different views of science, and especially medical science. The first tells us that science is a method of solving problems that is independent of the scientist; the second argues that the problems scientists tackle depend on their parents. The Nobel laureate believes in objective scientific truth; the Nazi is convinced that truth depends on one's subjective view of the world (*Weltan-schauung*). The first argument holds that science is value-free, the second that scientific truth is a social construct, a fiction, as it were. The belief of Albert Szent-Györgyi was shared by most medical scientists of the nineteenth century. Science, they were convinced, is indeed value-free, even if its consequences are caught in the tangle of time. The equation $pV = nRT$ describes the behavior of gases in hell or high water. There are, of course, notable exceptions, among them William James, who believed both in the spirit world and in objective science. He remained more skeptical of science than of the soul. James argued in an early chapter of his eloquent textbook *Psychology* (1901) that belief in reductionist science was a form of "spiritual chloroform. Better to live on the ragged edge, better to gnaw the file forever." Well, life on the ragged edge may be useful for the poet or philosopher, but not the scientist. As Auden explained, poetry is not science; what the scientist knows does not know him. Reductionists agree: a carbon atom knows neither reform nor chloroform. But James the half poet half believed in the mind of inanimate objects and therefore remained racked on the jagged edge of doubt. On the penultimate page of his two-volume treatise he was still gnawing the file between Lamarck and Darwin, nature and nurture, Christ and the chromosome. Yes, August Weismann had disproved the inheritance of acquired characteristics, but on the other hand . . .

These days it looks as if Weismann and his immutable chromosomes are going to have their way, and few can look forward without qualms to that day when the encyclopedia of our genes is completed. Whether the news from the human genome project be good or bad, most of us do not really want to know the truth, the whole truth, and nothing but the truth in our DNA library. Who really wishes to know at the age of twenty whether he is likely to die of stroke at fifty? Who wants to know if the baby will grow up to be Forrest Gump? Much of what is written in our genes is bad news. Already, the telltale runs of DNA that spell out cystic fibrosis, Huntington's chorea, β-thalassemia, or familial colon cancer can be read in the entrails of our cells. The most complex forms of idiocy, palsy, or immunodeficiency result from simple errors of genetic spelling or punctuation. Substitute a letter in the genetic code, say G for an A in the DNA at codon 216, and you get the amino acid glycine instead of arginine in the enzyme adenosine deaminase. An ill-fated child with this substitution—snakebit in the gene, as we said of Elsie Venner—will suffer from severe combined immunodeficiency (SCID) and be unable to cope with infections. Of course, not all the typographical errors that mar the page proofs of our genome lead to severe diseases like SCID or Alzheimer's. Most mistakes in the genome are innocuous and are destined to remain unnoticed on an uncut page of the finished volume. But most of us are afraid of what's written in that book.

The facts of life, just the facts, ma'am, will make few of us entirely happy. We tend to prefer the fancy music of hope to the plain speech of fact. That preference was spelled out in deft fashion by Dr. Oliver Wendell Holmes in his poem "The Coming Era":

> *Optics will claim the wandering eye of fancy,*
>   *Physics will grasp imagination's wings—*
> *Plain fact exorcise fiction's necromancy*
>   *The workshop hammer where the minstrel sings.*
>
> *So speak in solemn tomes our youthful sages,*
>   *Patient, severe, laborious, slow, exact,*
> *As o'er creation's protoplasmic pages*
>   *They browse and munch the thistle crops of fact.*

Dr. Holmes's warning that physics will grasp imagination's wing owes no small debt to Keats's "Lamia," with its warning that "philosophy will clip an Angel's wings," while his "thistle crop of fact" is a fancy version of Keats's reduction of taxonomy to "the dull catalogue of common things." Holmes and Keats, nineteenth-century poet-doctors, feared that in the coming era the facts of science would replace the insights of poetry. Worse yet, the Romantics were afraid that the adoption of scientific habits—patient, severe, laborious, slow, exact—would destroy not only esthetics but ethics as well. Poets of the last century preached that belief in poetry was an aspect of morals and for over a century their cultures agreed: English schoolboys learned from Keats that all one needed to know was that "beauty is truth, truth beauty" while most American children prayed with Holmes to "build me more stately mansions, O my soul!" But nowadays, as our violent century sputters to the millennium, as gun-toting tots spill out of schoolyards to the amplified doggerel of misogynist war chants, belief in the Romantic equation of ethics with esthetics seems like geriatric nostalgia. Unfortunately, our cacophonous avant-garde is no more encouraging than our lowlife. The postmodernist high jinks of our time ought to make anyone nostalgic for a golden age of poems that rhyme, paintings with figures in them, and operas with tunes to sing, nostalgic for a preindustrial age of sweetness and light, truth and beauty, *Dichtung und Warheit*, nostalgic for the age of, say, Keats and Goethe.

But no amount of Goethe or Schiller kept the most bookish nations of Europe from committing crimes past believing: in the days of the storm troopers, schoolchildren and aging scholars were forced to scrub pavements with toothbrushes around the statues of Goethe and Schiller on Vienna's Ringstrasse; truth and beauty, *Dichtung und Warheit* went underground at mid-century. The lives of great men do not all remind us that we can make our lives sublime. On the contrary, they warn us that a rarified imagination or a fancy eye is no guarantee of moral vigor. The horror shows of the twentieth century have enjoyed the support of poets (Ezra Pound), men of letters (Gabriele D'Annunzio), musicians (Richard Strauss), metaphysicians (Martin Heidegger) and estheticians (George Santayana). Those minstrels of nostalgia—and the regimes they upheld—were big fans of fiction's necromancy. They were also enemies of Western science and its leveling laws. Pound and Santayana became émigrés from America, disenchanted, one presumes, with their countrymen's attention to the dull catalogue of common things. Santayana's story is the real caution here. George Santayana, a fellow Harvard scholar of Holmes's old age and author of the aptly named *The Last Puritan*, had found a home in Mussolini's Italy before and during World War II. In an adulatory memoir, Edmund Wilson recalls Santayana's evaluation of the Duce after the war: "Oh, the regime was splendid, I assure you!" The Harvard émigré was impressed by fascist efficiency, "virility," and all those uniforms. Wilson and Santayana shared contempt for the classless, ill-educated mob of GIs who had come to Europe. Bad genes, they would have said. Wilson also relates how Santayana gladly contributed a gold medal to Mussolini's Abyssinian war chest. The medal had been awarded him by a British philosophical society a few years earlier for his work on the Platonic ideal of beauty. The Italians returned it to Santayana with regret that the medal was of insufficient value; it had been cast in lead and gilded.

We might argue that the Romantic conflation of beauty with truth is a notion that can't pass the acid test either. Truth and beauty still haven't recovered from the beating they took in the 1940s. Indeed, when we look about us today, their places have been taken by New Age necromancers and the cult of grunge. Happily our youthful sages of the genome seem to be doing better than the trendies of the arts. In Holmes's phrase, "creation's protoplasmic pages" are yielding a rich crop of facts indeed. And there, among the thistles, one can find the tough roots of a new ethic. The moral lessons that science has painfully learned from our mid-century explosions appear in every aspect of the new biology. Abandoned by the fashionable, truth and beauty have found refuge in the pages of *Nature* and *Science*.

✻

On July 16, 1993, a compelling research article by Dean Hamer and his colleagues at the National Cancer Institute appeared in *Science*, reporting a novel genetic discovery. The scientists ended their five pages of detailed genetics with a note of caution so remarkable that it does credit to all of our science:

> Our work represents an early application of molecular linkage methods to a normal variation in human behavior. As the human genome project proceeds, it is likely that many such correlations will be discovered. We believe that it would be fundamentally unethical to use such information to try to assess or alter a person's current or future sexual orientation, either heterosexual or homosexual, or other normal attributes of human behavior.

Hamer's team had found compelling evidence that a small chunk of DNA on the X chromosome (termed Xq28) contained a gene associated with male homosexuality. The team first determined that there were increased rates of same-sex orientation in maternal uncles and male cousins of male homosexuals (the probands) but not in their fathers or paternal relatives (114 families). Since uncles and cousins were raised in separate households from the probands, but clearly shared with them segments of the family's X chromosome, Hamer et al. postulated that male homosexuality was due to genetic nature and not nurture, and that the candidate gene or genes was on the X (maternal) chromosome. They now used the powerful tools of modern molecular genetics to study the X chromosomes of 40 families in which there were two gay brothers and no indication of paternal transmission, pointing out that "the recent advances in human genome analysis, in particular the development of chromosomal

genetic maps that are densely populated with highly polymor-
phic markers, make it feasible to apply such methods to complex
traits, such as sexual orientation, even if these traits are influ-
enced by multiple genes, or environmental factors, or some com-
bination of these."

Using the same polymerase chain reaction (PCR) that became
the stuff of late-night television in the O. J. Simpson era, they
were able to map a series of five marker genes. The PCR technique, for the discovery of which the 1993 Nobel Prize in chemistry was awarded, permits millions of copies of DNA to be
made from the tiniest samples of blood. They found that 33 of
40 pairs of brothers shared a set of five marker genes; all were
located near the end of the long arm of the X chromosome.
Their formal linkage analysis gave an "LOD score of 4.0" which
translates to a 99.5 percent certainty that the q28 region at the
tip of the coiled X chromosome predisposes to gay behavior.

The article attracted national attention and a flood of correspondence; two of these letters deserve note. In one, two ge-
neticists from Brown and Harvard, on the basis of various
statistical arguments, concluded that Hamer's data were not as
"robust" as they could be. (This use of nineteenth-century fit-
ness rhetoric on the geneticist's part suggests that both genes
and gene hunters are locked in a Darwinian struggle for survival.) But lack of robust data was not the only reason these
critics wondered whether it would not have been prudent for
Hamer—and *Science*—to have withheld these "preliminary
data." They rightly pointed out that "given the increased fre-
quency of hate crimes directed against homosexuals it is fair and
literal to say that lives are at stake."

The most poignant response was that of Rochelle Diamond,
chair of the National Organization of Gay and Lesbian Scientists and Technical Professionals, of Pasadena. Diamond co-
gently summarized two possible consequences of the Hamer
study for gays and lesbians: "On the one hand, we are pleased
that there is now scientific evidence that sexual orientation has

an immutable component. On the other, this work raises the specter of various possibilities of screening for such components." Diamond pointed out that Hamer's data could be used to support gay and lesbian civil-rights cases on the basis of a "biological imperative." But she also reminded readers of possible misuses of science by zealots of social Darwinism and eugenics. "We are concerned," she wrote, "that, in the future, it may be possible to screen fetuses, allowing for termination of pregnancy on such a basis." Bravely, she argued for continued research into genetics, supporting "scientific freedom and the social responsibilities that go along with its discoveries. We believe that basic research such as Hamer et al.'s work should be pursued in order to further our understanding of how the universe works."

Diamond and her enlightened colleagues need moral and political support over a very long haul indeed. Scientist and layman alike must assure them that the thistles of fact—the genes of gender—don't stick in the craw of bigots. The fact that some behaviors have a genetic component ought to be a liberating rather than a limiting aspect of truth. Indeed, studies like Hamer's argue the case for proceeding with getting the facts, and just the facts, whether we like them or not.

At the end of this squalid era, what an upbeat enterprise the gene-hunt project has turned out to be! And how different in tone and feeling from the, literally, depressive views of those, like Edmund Wilson, who dominated the arts of our time. Here is how America's most eminent man of letters described American GIs in the postwar London of 1945: "These human amoebas were left to drift about in the back eddy of England. What had the war worked up to? Nothing—vacuity—these unintegrated human organisms with no training in directing themselves, with no strong impulses toward self-direction . . . Soon the globe will be known and a bore." Two decades later, he was still bored: "I told Malraux that life in America is *une espèce d'enfer,* that there was little to choose between us and the Soviet

Union" (1962). And again, "I find that I more and more feel a boredom with and scorn for the human race" (1968).

But when the secrets of our globe and of our genes are really known they will by no means be boring. We've already learned so much since those "human amoebas" returned from cleaning up a mess caused by the genetic pen pals of Pound and Santayana. Wilson's patrician prose—and gloomy scorn—ought to remind us that when the genome is completely deciphered, we'd better keep its secrets from misuse by those who are "bored" by the globe and its inhabitants. The failure of nerve at the end of World War II was a sorry replay of the one that Wilson hinted at in *Patriotic Gore*. And the divergence of social aims between sanguine scientist and saturnine belletrist has not advanced the cause of democracy in the age of DNA.

We could do worse than to heed Rochelle Diamond's meliorist plea that "now is the time to address the ethical questions surrounding the use of such information in advance, so that the ethics may evolve with the science instead of lagging behind, as often happens." The ethics *are* evolving, and Dr. Holmes offers us the standard, spelling it out in sentiments that have been carried in our species as long as the codons of the double helix.

> *Well, Time alone can lift the future's curtain,—*
> *Science may teach our children all she knows,*
> *But Love will kindle fresh young hearts, 't is certain*
> *And June will not forget her blushing rose.*
>
> *And, so, in spite of all that Time is bringing—*
> *Treasures of truth and miracles of art,*
> *Beauty and Love will keep the poet singing,*
> *And song still live, the science of the heart.*

As these verses show, Holmes is no Keats, but on the other hand, he *is* the one we should trust with the secrets we are about to decipher on "creation's protoplasmic pages." He wouldn't be bored at all.

15. WHATSOEVER WINDS
MAY BLOW

But it was at night, long after the family had gone to sleep, that my father's hardest work began. The telephone started ringing after midnight. I could hear it from my bedroom down the hall, and I could hear his voice, tired and muffled by sleep, asking for details, and then I could hear him hang up the phone in the dark; usually he would swear "Damnation," sometimes he was distressed enough to use flat-out "Damn it," or worse, "Damn"; rarely did I hear him say, in total fury, "God Damn it." Then I could hear him heave out of bed, the sounds of dressing, lights in the hall, and then his steps down the back stairs, out in the yard and into the car, and off on a house call. This happened every night at least once, sometimes three or four times.

—Lewis Thomas, *The Youngest Science*, 1983

Abigail Thomas read this selection from her father's work on the occasion of the first Lewis Thomas Prize ceremony in 1993. Fittingly enough, plucky, ailing Lewis Thomas was the first recipient of the award given by Rockefeller University which in his name "seeks to honor that rare individual in whom the two cultures of science and art are combined"—to quote the terms of the prize. Lewis Thomas died six months later.

The audience gathered that spring afternoon included former students and residents, colleagues, family, friends, and the doyens of New York art and science. What was striking, if unsurprising, was the presence of doctors—and the sons and daughters of doctors. The passage from *The Youngest Science* that Abigail Thomas was reading described the life of Lewis Thomas's own father, a busy practitioner in Flushing, New York, in the 1930s. *The Youngest Science* is a limpid autobiography that connects medicine with literature and brings us into the era of DNA. Since Abigail Thomas is herself a writer whose first book of short stories was to appear in the summer of 1994, many in the audience must have been reminded of other familial bonds between the medical and literary vocations. Indeed, were we to ask what Ernest Hemingway had in common with Oscar Wilde, Sinclair Lewis with Marcel Proust, Adrienne Rich with Friedrich Schiller, John O'Hara with Gustave Flaubert, and Michel Foucault with W. H. Auden, we would answer that they were all the children of doctors. Judging from this list, only some children ever forgive their fathers.

In the course of that ceremony other family ties came to mind. The first president of the Rockefeller Institute, which only recently became a university, was Simon Flexner. Flexner was a distinguished microbiologist whose name now survives as that of the dysentery bacillus (*S. flexneri*). In his lifetime he became infamous as a fictional character; Sinclair Lewis depicts him in *Arrowsmith* as the smarmy director of the McGurk Institute for Medical Research. No wonder! Paul de Kruif, the unacknowledged co-author of *Arrowsmith*, had been dismissed by Flexner in 1923 from the Rockefeller Institute for falsified claims and publicity seeking. De Kruif had written a trendy exposé of the medical establishment for the *Century* magazine under the anonymous signature of K____, M.D. Unfortunately, he had quit medical school to obtain a Ph.D. in bacteriology and so his "inside" confession was more fiction than fact. But de Kruif was more than a self-destructive iconoclast. As a young researcher, he had performed experiments that might have put him in position to discover that DNA was the "transforming principle" of the rough-to-smooth transformation of pneumococcus, a line of investigation that eventually proved crucial to the Flowering of DNA. But Flexner put a stop to de Kruif's career as a microbe hunter. It is therefore no surprise that de Kruif failed to forgive his scientific father.

In turn, Simon Flexner was far more generous to *his* father in science, William Henry Welch. Not only did Flexner entitle the biography of his mentor *William Henry Welch and the Heroic Age of American Medicine*, but his filial glow extended to William Welch's father, a practitioner in Litchfield County, Connecticut, in the 1850s:

> The doctor was always detained by patients who came late and stayed long, while he advised them not only on health but on crops, politics, family affairs, manufactures and the probable state of the weather. . . . It was usually almost dark before the doctor started out with a well-filled lantern slung underneath the buggy and a Dalmatian dog running at the horse's heels. . . . Late passers-by would see a lantern swinging low, making crazy shadows, and then catch a glimpse of a flowing beard as the doctor rushed behind one of his powerful horses. Often the doctor would be asleep as he travelled at breakneck speed, but . . . if he were not asleep, he could hardly resist stopping to speak to every passer-by he met, for all in the community were his patients and his friends. These conversations, usually long and intimate, were sometimes interrupted by his friend's asking him how much he owed for past medical services. Such a question never failed to fluster William Wickham Welch. "Oh, never mind now; we are in a hurry," he would reply as he whipped up his horse.

Litchfield in 1850 and Flushing in 1930 weren't all that different when it came to the remedies that doctors could offer their patients. Neither the sanitary nor the bacteriological revolution had changed things much at the bedside. One could have said before World War II what Dr. Holmes said before the Civil War: "If the whole materia medica, as now used, could be sunk to the bottom,—it would be the better for mankind and all the worse for the fishes." Insulin, vitamins, and local anesthetics had been introduced, but as he trudged out at late at night with his "God Damn," Dr. Thomas had little more of use in that black bag than had Dr. Welch eighty years before.

As the program continued that spring afternoon with another of Lewis Thomas's daughters, Eliza Thomas, playing the *andante grazioso* of Mozart's A major piano sonata K. 331, many in the audience must have felt a strong resonance between that passage from *The Youngest Science* and their own childhood memories. It was the era, to use Thomas's phrase, when medicine was turning into a science—at least at places like the Rockefeller Institute—but when the old art was still in place. I, too, had been awakened by late-night or early-morning calls to hear my father grumbling out of bed in response to real or imagined emergencies. Black bag in hand, doctors of my father's generation, as of generations before, went out into the cold night to dispense a little science and much art after they had muttered their God Damn. They sure weren't whistling Mozart. My father died on one of those house calls.

Sinclair Lewis knew that sort of life and put the best of his father's ideals into Martin Arrowsmith.

> Mary was a child of seven or eight. Martin found her lips and fingertips blue, but in her face no flush . . . Martin worried as he took out his clinical thermometer and gave it a professional shake It was, he decided, laryngeal croup or diphtheria. Probably diphtheria . . . He would use diphtheria antitoxin. He regained confidence. He thanked the god of science for antitoxin and for the gas motor. It was, he decided, a Race with Death. "I'm going to do it—going to pull it off and save that poor kid!" he rejoiced.

Sinclair Lewis's conflation of the romance of medicine with a romantic genre (The Race with Death) is not unique in the annals of doctor's stories. If memory serves, Goethe told the tale first in *Der Erlkönig*. The child in the poem dies on the way to the doctor, the race is lost. But in Sinclair Lewis's novel, medical knowledge—science, not art alone—wins the race. Martin Arrowsmith could be said to have been Peter Medawar's sanguine meliorist in action, "one who believes that the world can be improved by finding out what is wrong with it and then taking steps to put it right."

Hemingway also honored the meliorism of medicine in his story "Indian Camp." He describes a tough breech delivery that his father made on the Upper Peninsula of Michigan:

> "Those must boil," he said, and began to soak his hands in the basin of hot water with a cake of soap he had brought from the camp. Nick watched his father's hands scrubbing each other with the soap. . . . Nick held the basin for his father. It all took a long time. . . . His father picked the baby up and slapped it to make it breathe and handed it to the old woman. "See, it's a boy, Nick," he said. "How do you like being an interne?"

Flaubert described *his* father—a distinguished practitioner of Rouen—in the guise of the fictional Dr. Larivière in Madame Bovary as one who:

> cherishing their art with a fanatical love, exercised it with enthusiasm and wisdom. . . . Disdainful of honors, of titles, and of academies, hospitable, generous, fatherly to the poor, and practicing virtue without believing in it, he would almost have passed for a saint if the keenness of his intellect had not caused him to be feared as a demon.

The audience gathered at Rockefeller University was certainly not disdainful of honors, titles, or academies. But if keenness of intellect was widespread, so was the practice of virtue. Some of these medical scientists might pass as temporal saints who had fulfilled the dreams of sanitarians and reformers alike to accomplish God's work on earth. Unlike those of the deity, however, the miracles of medical science are reproducible. Some of those in the auditorium had presided over the Flowering of DNA and lived to see it bear fruit. At that moment, laboratories up and down the East River were splicing tumor suppressor genes into cancer cells to quell their growth.

It's been a long journey from the black-bag days of our fathers to music and prizes at Rockefeller, but the motives of the profession seem constant. Lewis Thomas and his father had both spent their lives pursuing Peter Medawar's definition of the meliorist faith, "finding out what is wrong and then taking steps to put it right." That coincidence of science and art by the East River also fulfilled the Puritan charge that its anointed become "the herald of light and the bearer of love." Jonathan Edwards prefaced the biography of *his* father in learning, John Winthrop, with Cicero's epigraph *Quicunque Venti Erunt, Ars Nostra Certe Non Aberunt* (Whatever Winds May Blow, Our Art Will Never Pass Away). A glimpse around that audience, young and old alike, was reassuring: Greek and Barbarian, Jew and Gentile as Holmes had it in Paris; but now also men and women; Muslim and Hindu; white, brown, black, and yellow. Not quite what Edwards would have had in mind, but no matter. The molecular revolution seemed in good hands. *Quicunque Venti Erunt, Ars Nostra Certe Non Aberunt.*

Torsten Wiesel, the gentle Nobel laureate who succeeded David Baltimore as president of Rockefeller University, next presented the prize to Lewis Thomas, who, confined to a wheelchair by illness, apologized to the audience for "not rising to the occasion." I was reminded of a telephone call I had made to him a while ago. "How are you doing?" I had asked, before going on to the business end of our conversation. "So," he replied. "What do you mean by 'so'?" I asked. "Well," said Thomas. "In my family, there were only three ways of answering that question of yours. If things were going along splendidly, you'd answer 'fine.' If there were a bit of trouble around, you'd say 'so-so.' Well, right now, I'm 'so.' "

Lewis Thomas's "so" had been everyone else's "fine." Ailing on and off for a decade, this most *grazioso* of doctor-writers was the source of innumerable new essays, reviews, and addresses, published two volumes, and remained living proof that it is possible for wit and erudition to coexist in the presence of poetry. Stephen Jay Gould, in his review of *The Youngest Science*, pointed out that Thomas's modest claims for medical science have always been allied to a fondness for its art. Gould was sure that what modern medicine most needed was an army of Lewis Thomas clones. I was sure that Thomas may have been the one among us who best combined George Eliot's charge to combine intellectual conquest with social good. Like Peter Medawar—one of his best friends—he was of sanguine temperament.

❊

As the citation was read, I remembered the moment that Lewis Thomas asked me to be his chief resident at Bellevue. I was still deciding whether to follow my father into practice or move on to an academic career in science. When Dr. Thomas told me what academic salaries were like in the late 1950s, my impertinent younger self quoted, in dismay: "What is science but the absence of prejudice in the presence of money?" "Henry James," said Lewis Thomas, "from *The Golden Bowl*, chapter one." He went on, "All right then, you won't earn very much but you'll have a lot of fun in the lab and time to read. My dad never did have much time." In the event, I have remained at NYU-Bellevue ever since.

Ars Nostra Certe Non Aberunt. One had that feeling about those two institutions on the East River, NYU-Bellevue and Rockefeller University. I recalled a sparkling day earlier that year when a group of us had listened to Bill Clinton's inaugural speech thirty blocks downriver.

My fellow citizens, today we celebrate the mystery of American renewal. This ceremony is held in the depth of winter, but by the words we speak and the faces we show the world, we force the spring.

At noon on inauguration day at Bellevue Hospital, in the empty patients' lounge, with the new President's face flickering from a vandalized TV screen, the metaphor itself wasn't entirely forced. On that clear day the corner lounge was filled with sunlight and yielded splendid views. Much of Manhattan was visible from the sixteenth floor of our hospital tower on the East River: the Chrysler and Empire State buildings, the UN, the megaliths of midtown, the apartment towers flanking the Queensboro Bridge. Directly under the riverside windows were a busy heliport and a flag-bedecked restaurant. White puffs trailed from tugs on the river. No slums, no squalor, no crime visible from that height.

That sunlit municipal hospital of 1993 was a far cry from the tatty red-brick almshouse of 1878 in which William Henry Welch had established the first pathology laboratory in this country. His friend Henry C. Coe was concerned: "I felt instinctively that he was wasted at Bellevue and was destined to have a larger circle of hearers." He needn't have worried. Welch went on to become one of the "Four Doctors" who put Johns Hopkins on the medical map, established laboratory medicine in the United States as a discipline, and installed his student Simon Flexner at the head of the institute that Welch had persuaded Rockefeller to fund. By 1908 it was as America's preeminent medical scientist that he introduced his teacher, Robert Koch, at that dinner with Andrew Carnegie: *Lebe hoch, Robert Koch!*

Welch had worked in the old red-brick structure, and there have been other incarnations of Bellevue Hospital and its medical school. But what Oliver Wendell Holmes said of the old Harvard Medical School tenement has been true over Bellevue's history as well: "This temple of learning is not surrounded by the mansions of the great and the wealthy. No stately avenues lead up to its facades and porticoes. I have sometimes felt, when convoying a distinguished stranger through its precincts to its door, that he might question whether star-eyed Science had not missed her way when she found herself in this not too attractive locality."

New York has built the closest thing possible these days to an alabaster city fit for star-eyed Science: a high-rise of concrete and steel. That new Bellevue is a visible monument to the meliorist tradition in New York, combining, as it were, the intellectual aim of conquering disease with the social goal of treating the poor. Over the years the place has attracted innovative doctors like William Welch to work there "long enough for Bellevue to go to his head and stay there, as it does to the minds of most people who work in that place for great stretches." Those words of Lewis Thomas could apply to another young Bellevue doctor, named Maclyn McCarty, who went up to Rockefeller Institute and—with Colin MacLeod and Oswald Avery—performed the critical experiments which showed that the "transforming principle" was pure DNA. It could be said that the Flowering of DNA began by the East River, but that would be bragging.

It was believed a generation ago when the "new" Bellevue was on the drawing board that social planning and public expenditure could effect a sort of American renewal in health. Robert Wagner and John Vliet Lindsay, liberal Democratic and Republican mayors of our city, had made our hospital possible in 1973. In return, Lewis Thomas, who was not only chief of medicine at NYU-Bellevue but a member of the planning committee for the new structure, celebrated our hospital as an "immense institutional model of the human universe." It all seems a century ago. These days our universe, like its model, contains crack and AIDS and drug-resistant tuberculosis.

In the patients' lounge on Clinton's inauguration day, two

pajama-clad junkies had quickly stamped out their cigarillos on the floor and left. The smell of Phillies Blunts remained and a pile of butts was underfoot, as the new President spoke from an erratic screen:

> Now the sights and sounds of this ceremony are broadcast instantaneously to billions around the world. Communications and commerce are global, investment is mobile, technology is almost magical, and ambition for a better life is now universal.

Among the "billions around the world" were the patients of the sixteenth floor at Bellevue. And among those patients were crack addicts, chronic alcoholics, abandoned pensioners, dazed drifters, dismissed domestics, the unemployed, and the illegals. Many had spent the New Year sleeping in doorways or on subway gratings. Now they were housed in clean two- or four-bed sickrooms with white sheets and shining beds. Empty lunch trays were stacked on carts. They had found a temporary home at Bellevue, which fulfills for our city the charge of Robert Frost: "Home is the place where when you have to go there / They have to take you in."

Above each bed was a large television set which had presumably remained unvandalized because it was unreachable. Each set showed pictures of the President and most of the patients lay flat in bed to listen to his words. Against the doorways, also listening to the President, leaned nurses, nurse's aides, kitchen help, janitors, and cops. Cops and more cops: transit and hospital cops in the hall, correction cops from Rikers Island—the city prison—in the patients' rooms.

Bellevue employs 5,500 people and seems to be under almost permanent occupation by a gun-toting brigade of police. A platoon of cops is required for each of three shifts a day to man the prison ward, another platoon or two to man the "outposts" when a prisoner is too sick to be housed on the prison ward or when it is full. One platoon transfers prisoners in and out of lorries and another crew in blue seems to be employed exclusively in shuttling coffee up and down the elevators. On inauguration day, the cops, coffee in hand, stood cheek by jowl with their prisoners, listening to the President. House-staff doctors stood in clusters by the door, janitors watched from beside pails. Looking at the assembled crew from our vantage point in the lounge, it was difficult to know what the global nature of communication and commerce, the mobility of investment, or the magic of technology meant to the audience on the sixteenth floor. An ambition for a better life? Who would not wish for a life better than that of the sick and poor in a city hospital? Clinton had gone on:

> But when most people are working harder for less, when others cannot work at all, when the cost of health care devastates families and threatens to bankrupt our enterprises great and small, when the fear of crime robs law-abiding citizens of their freedom, and when millions of poor children cannot even imagine the lives we are calling them to lead, we have not made change our friend.

Most of the patients at Bellevue were not working harder for less; they were not working at all. Many have never worked. As many have committed crime as have been its victims. Indeed, on one or another tally sheet, they have all been counted as victims. Losers in the economic war, they have not had their enterprises bankrupted by health care, nor have they been devastated by its cost. Our city may, however, have been hurt by expense: Bellevue spends $370 million a year on 20,000 inpatients, 90,000 emergency visits, and 360,000 outpatient visits. Only 3 percent of our patients have paid for their own care, and private insurance for only 14 percent more. The rest comes from the public purse: $19 million from the city's taxes alone. Illegal aliens—an estimated one fifth of our admissions—are paid from Medicaid, part of the 64 percent of our hospital's income that derives from that source. Our taxes pay for nurses and medicines, CAT scans and bypass surgery, an AIDS ward and a gym, a school for disturbed children, an elaborate dietary and social work establishment, several ICUs, and the latest in microsurgery. It could indeed be argued that good medical care in a hospital is one of the few reliable services New York City has provided for its poor. Moreover, were many of these medical services not pro bono, their costs would be even higher than $370 million a year. But those who have worked here all their lives remain convinced that, rich or poor, good medicine is like Frost's idea of home: "Something you somehow haven't to deserve." The new President sounded his trumpet of the American dream of progress: "There is nothing wrong with America that cannot be cured by what is right in America."

What's wrong with America is not hard to document at Bellevue. As Andy Logan—the scribe of New York—has pointed out, our city has over 10 percent unemployment; one million are on welfare and two thousand New Yorkers are murdered each year. To our hospital are brought the murderers, the crazed, the violent, the abused, the newborn rescued from trash cans, the assaulted jogger, the homeless derelict set on fire in the subways. To our doors are also brought women who have given birth in taxis, women whose children are said to have been born out of gridlock. In our libertarian hospital, unrestrained patients—the mad, the angry, the tubercular—wander the corridors at will; many of them cannot or will not read the prohibitory notices. The stairways are littered with syringes, condoms, and crack vials. One of our young pathologists was recently stabbed to death in her office while preparing slides for a teaching conference. And Dr. Holmes thought that Harvard was no fit home for star-eyed Science!

When middle-class visitors come to Bellevue they are dazed by the noise and tumult. The racial mix, what David Dinkins called "the gorgeous mosaic," disturbs them, the crowded lobby is threatening, the waiting room is strange and confusing. The costumes are warlike and the place is thronged by what adolescent psychiatrists call dudes with an attitude. "It's like practicing medicine in a subway," the house staff complain. "It's a squalid, old-fashioned city hospital," the visitors tell us. But the squalor is only skin-deep.

What is right in America is the unbroken compact our city has kept with its poor for 250 years. Bellevue is, indeed, an old-fashioned city hospital, but its doctors practice newfangled medicine. The physicians of Bellevue and NYU have included William Gorgas and Walter Reed, Austin Flint and Stephen Smith, Emily Blackwell and Josephine Baker, William Welch and Lewis Thomas. Pathology, psychiatry, pediatrics, and pulmonology got their municipal start here; and in a room where my electron microscope now sits, Dickinson Richards and André Cournand of Columbia won the Nobel Prize for cardiac catheterization. Fit or not, Bellevue has been the home of star-eyed Science.

Today, as for many generations, our house officers number among the most desirable of medical graduates. The poorest immigrant from Hong Kong will receive a more painstaking workup than the owner of the Peninsula Hotel in Kowloon. The government agrees. When the President of the United States visits New York City, Bellevue goes on standby as the primary receiving hospital in case of an emergency. Not only officials, but the surly warriors who arrive with the battle wounds of street violence and drug addiction are cared for by their brothers and sisters who have made health care their profession. The medicines dripping into the veins of our patients on the sixteenth floor are as carefully monitored as those in the richest hospital in the land. The latest gadgets of diagnosis gleam from the cupboard. What Lewis Thomas said of Bellevue a generation ago stands true today, "If I were to be taken sick in a taxicab

with something serious or struck down in a New York street, I
would want to be taken to Bellevue." *Ars Nostra Certe Non
Aberunt* indeed.

✳

Those Bellevue recollections were replaced by others as Abigail
Thomas read more of her father's work at Rockefeller University: Some of those passages seemed like prose poems on the
Great Chain of Being. One was reminded that urban ills and
social squalor do not define the human condition. Thomas believed that our nature was wired for self-improvement. Looking
around at that audience of doctors, scholars, readers, it was easy
to agree. It seemed clear that we formed a sort of "local hill, or
hive, or nest, or flight," a grouping of social animals, that Lewis
Thomas likened to the parts of a human brain:

> Come to think of it, our minds are already interconnected, in
> increasingly dense and complex circuits and relays; we are
> already gathering and exchanging information as incessantly
> as the ants . . . we exchange information, pass it around to
> each other, store it, retrieve it, process it. If we keep at it, we
> will discover, bit by bit, how the system works, and then,
> perhaps as a kind of footnote, how we fit in.

Thomas wrote that passage in an address, "Adaptive Aspects of
Inflammation," given at a meeting organized by a group of
young scientists who began a club to study inflammation. The
symposium was held in June 1970, and it marked the emergence
of Lewis Thomas as a man of letters.

Between his return from World War II in 1946 and that piece
of writing in 1970, Thomas had been the model of the gifted,
productive, laboratory-based academic physician and adminis-
trator. He had moved from strength to strength as professor,
department head, and dean—from Tulane to Minnesota to NYU
and to Yale. He had discovered heterologous antibodies in viral

pneumonia and shown that the generalized Shwartzman reaction would not proceed without white cells or blood clots. He discovered that foreign proteases (for example, the meat tenderizer, papain) or native ferments released by an excess of vitamin A caused the breakdown of connective tissue. Cortisone was protective against such insults. More importantly, it was Thomas who first suggested that the same lymphocytes that recognize and attack foreign, transplanted tissue were responsible for the immune surveillance of cancer cells. A sterling performance in research!

Of equal sparkle was his role as a medical educator. At each school he graced, he left behind a group of physician-scientists who were not only brought into research by him but whose work was to be marked by the kind of elegant, heuristic flair that Thomas expected: the names of Baruj Benacerraf, Robert Good, Jonathan Uhr, Philip Patterson, H. Sherwood Lawrence, Edward Franklin, John David, Emil Gottschlich, Stuart Schlossman, R. T. McCluskey, Jeanette Thorbecke, and Chandler Stetson come immediately to mind. The glittering prizes—including a Nobel—came easily to this group. He trained dozens of eminent clinicians as well: at NYU he was known as the "Pied Piper of Bellevue." In the days of the old red-brick hospital, he charmed many of us into an academic or clinical career under conditions that few dockworkers would tolerate—and for about twenty-five dollars a month.

And then came the day that Lewis Thomas delivered his eloquent speech on inflammation at Brook Lodge. The organizers had asked me to invite him to give the after-dinner speech of the symposium. It therefore fell on me to introduce my former chief and after I paid the usual, fumbling tribute, Lew mounted the podium, murmured, "Thank you, I think," and proceeded to launch the most splendid literary career of any physician since Anton Chekhov. Despite the generous dinner, despite the warm June night of 1970, the somnolent inflammation boffins were knocked out of their seats. Accustomed to the passive voice of

dreary fact, they heard instead the active buzz of a poet thinking. In the course of that talk, Thomas made more sense of
inflammation in fifty minutes of elegant prose than had prolix lecturers on endotoxin or macrophages in the preceding
sixteen hours. It was a reassuring test of the hypothesis that if
one has something to say, it can be said in English. The talk—
written and delivered with great humor—proved not only that
twentieth-century science was a fit subject for literature but
that the Youngest Science of medicine had found its freshest
voice. The talk was printed, someone brought it to the attention
of Franz Ingelfinger—editor of the *New England Journal of
Medicine*—and Thomas began his career as author of "Notes of
a Biology Watcher." Thanks to Elisabeth Sifton, then an editor
at The Viking Press, those marvelous, bimonthly essays were
soon collected into *The Lives of a Cell*, the volume became a
best-seller and won a National Book Award—and the rest is
history.

Thomas's inflammation essay touched on almost every theme
that he later elaborated in his quarter century of literary performance. He began by explaining to us that were it not for the
phenomenon of inflammation—the capacity of self to reject
nonself—if there "were no mechanism around to counter the
drift toward unity, we might end up in fact as a single organism,
with all kinds of unworkable problems." Thomas also revealed
himself as the ultimate optimist of the human condition: "I take
it in faith that we are all better off as individuals with individual
cells, to the limited extent that individuality, in this sense, really
exists."

※

Another reading from Abigail Thomas was followed by a quar-
tet of gifted professionals playing Bach's "Art of the Fugue."
As that most didactic of masterpieces filled the round hall with
counterpoint, one was reminded of Thomas's suggestion that if
we needed a language to communicate with unknown creatures

out in space he "would vote for Bach, all of Bach streamed out into space over and over again. We would be bragging of course, but it is surely excusable to put the best possible face on at the beginning of such an acquaintance. We can tell the harder truths later."

What a broad view of humankind Thomas embraced: "We are, after all, a kind of single creature, if you take a long enough view of us and forget about time. We began in lightning, methane and cyanide or in some similar explosive way . . ." This immediate extrapolation to a very long view exasperated many of his co-workers over the years; when one's buffer had gone awry, or one's patient's potassium was dropping, or one needed more space to work, it was discouraging to be told that such problems were trivial in comparison to secrets of the universe. "I went in to Lew to ask if I could have an extra technician," a young assistant professor told me at the time. "He talked to me for about an hour about Teilhard de Chardin and I came away feeling great. I don't think I got the tech!" But with good nature, practical enthusiasm, and acute intelligence, Thomas addressed the mundane as neatly as the infinite, e.g.: "The dog skin reacting to the dog tick is an excellent illustration of the destruction of one's own tissues by one's own polymorphonuclear leukocytes."

A mind that extended from the alternative pathway of complement activation (the dog-tick mechanism) to the music of Bach was no small piece of evolutionary change! Sending Bach may indeed be bragging, and using Lewis Thomas as the model genome for a generation of humane physicians would probably constitute bragging of a similar order. But that afternoon it appeared that the essence of a learned profession, a profession that spreads its wings from night calls in Flushing to Bach at the Rockefeller, was to provide a space in which the generous aspects of its science can thrive together with its art. As Bach flowed over that audience, the young and the old, those doctors, their children and grandchildren, the art and the science were joined for a while in seamless conjunction. The efflorescent Baroque and the Flowering of DNA seemed to have come together as naturally as the strands of a gene. Thomas had worried about the cloning of genes at a time when the human genome project promised to become nothing more than routine engineering:

> I have an alternative suggestion. Set cloning aside and don't try it. Instead go in the other direction. Look for ways to get mutations more quickly, new variety, different songs. Fiddle around, if you must fiddle, but never with ways to keep things the same, no matter who, not even yourself. Heaven, somewhere ahead, has got to be a change.

Change or not, as Auden said of Yeats, now that Thomas is dead he has become his readers. Unlike Yeats, however, who dabbled in the occult, Thomas lives on in star-eyed Science. Thomas made several predictions that were smack on, even before more rigorous work in the lab confirmed how right he was. The immune surveillance of tumor cells is only one example, but it was the example Peter Medawar had in mind when he said of Thomas that there has been no one like him since Dr. Oliver Wendell Holmes. Were Thomas to have lived as long as Holmes, he might look back on immune surveillance as did Holmes on the fiftieth anniversary of his announcement of the contagiousness of puerperal fever:

> I thought I had proved my point and set the question of the private pestilence, as I called it, at rest "for good and all." . . . I do know that others cried out with all their might against this terrible evil before I did and I gave them full credit for it. But I think I shrieked louder and longer than any of them and I am pleased to remember that I took my ground on the existing evidence before the little army of microbes was marched up to support my position.

Well, before the little army of genes was marched up to support Thomas's position, before we could perform recombinant tricks with DNA vectors, Thomas had a hunch of how to fulfill Emerson's prediction that a chemist of our century might take "protoplasm or mix his hydrogen, oxygen, and carbon, and make an animalcule incontestably swimming and jumping before my eyes." Thomas knew that

> you can take unimagined liberties with amoebae: you can separate out the membranes, cytoplasm, and nuclei of amoebae, keep these bits alive, and then reassemble them like the part of different clocks, with one donor's membrane, another's nucleus, and the cytoplasm of a third, and the final animal swims about and feeds as though made in heaven.

Those amoebae dancing in the dish, teased apart and reassembled, are only some of the counters in the game of molecular biology. These days we toy with genes and cell parts snatched from fruit fly and sea snail, squid nerve and sponge cell, microbe and worm. No link in the Great Chain of Being has been left unexamined. And as fast as prudence would allow, the stuff of the lab has flowed into the clinic; the game after all is played for mortal stakes. Emerson would have agreed that "the day had arrived when the human race might be trusted with a new degree of power, and its immense responsibility; for these steps [are] only a hint of an advanced frontier supported by an advancing race behind it."

❊

The results of the sanitarian, bacteriological, and biological revolutions speak for themselves: whereas the death rate in New York City in 1845 was 27.3 per thousand, by 1992 it had dropped to 8.5. That aspect of God's work on earth was not accomplished by the pious or mesmeric; our science has been busy with deed not creed. From Samuel Gridley Howe to Eliz-

abeth Blackwell, from Oliver Wendell Holmes to William
Henry Welch, from the transforming principle to the double
helix, to the gene therapy of today, our revolutions have been
fueled by the spirit of meliorist reform. Whatever else our own
mean century has wrought, it has witnessed the Flowering of
DNA, which has given us the power to find out what goes
wrong in a sick body and to take steps to put it right. As for
the body politic, why, in the words of Stephen Sondheim's *Fol-
lies* girl, we've been through Herbert and J. Edgar Hoover!

Reductionist, scientific medicine may still be helpless in the
face of metastatic cancer, AIDS—or even chronic backache. And
the rude machines of medical progress may have defeated, in
part, the pastoral role of the family doctor. But that is no reason
to settle for magic potions or transcendental meditation. There
is no homeopathic, Ayurvedic, or New Age practice that can
prevent pandemics of plague, protect the earth from decay or
pollution, or prolong the life of a tot with a congenital hole in
its heart. When Kurds, Somalis, or Bosnians suffer from the
revival of traditional tribalism, they do not call for shamans or
homeopaths, but the plasma and antibiotics of Médecins sans
Frontières. The cholera and dysentery epidemics of Rwanda
were quelled by salt, potassium, and antimicrobials from stores
kept by the medical services of the American and French military. When the Ebola virus threatens the world from Zaire, aid
comes not from herbalists or chiropractors, but from the CDC
in Atlanta. Like Peter Medawar, those of us of sanguine temperament believe that many of our social hurts will yield with
time to reason or fall, like slavery, to force. Writing on the occasion of another inauguration, that of Abraham Lincoln, a sanguine James Russell Lowell spelled out the meliorist faith. He
was not only speaking of slavery, but spelling out an American
dream:

> The encroachments of slavery upon our national policy have
> been like those of a glacier in a Swiss valley. Inch by inch,

the huge dragon with its glittering scales and crests of ice coils itself onward, an anachronism of summer, the relics of a by-gone world where such monsters swarmed. But it has its limit, the silent arrows of the sun are still, as of old, fatal to the frosty Python. Geology tells us that such enormous devas-tators once covered the face of the earth, but the benignant sunlight of heaven touched them, they faded silently, leaving no trace, but here and there the scratches of their talons, and the gnawed boulders scattered where they made their lair. We have entire faith in the benignant influence of Truth, the sun-light of the moral world, and believe that slavery, like other worn-out systems, will melt gradually before it.

ACKNOWLEDGMENTS

I owe not only the title of this book to my wife, Ann, but also many of the themes it addresses. Without her own interests, fueled by work at the New-York Historical Society, I would not have become as engaged by nineteenth-century American civilization as is the obvious case. My agent, Gloria Loomis, and my editor, Elisabeth Sifton, have again helped me to join form to function in the architecture of this book. To Ms. Sifton, especially, belongs much of the credit for turning an essayist into a writer. Several of the themes in this book have been addressed in the monthly essays published by *MD* magazine in the years 1991–94 when I served as its editor-in-chief. I should like to thank my colleagues at that magazine, especially David Fisher, Helen Smith, Merrill Cason, John Shoemaker, and Terry Fagan, for their assistance, suggestions, and companionship. In very different settings, portions of this material appeared in the form of critical essays in *The New Republic*, *The Yale Review*, and *The New Criterion*. My other special thanks go to the extensive joint library of the Marine Biological Laboratory and the Woods Hole Oceanographic Institution, over which Cathy Norton now presides. That library is as much of a national treasure as the laboratories it supports. I am also indebted to the well-situated private library of Mme Arlette Gaillet on the Quai Bourbon in Paris, where much of my writing is done each year and where I have attempted to translate Baudelaire. Since many sections of this book are based on published volumes of letters and memoirs, I would also like to acknowledge the help of several book sellers of Cape Cod who have permitted me to stock my own library of American authors. I am very grateful for the assistance—and existence—of the Market Bookshop and Falmouth Books of Falmouth; Isaiah Thomas of Cotuit and Parnassus Books of Yarmouthport.

I would also like to thank my colleagues at New York University Medical Center who have had to cope with a doctor hunting for belletristic material amid laboratory and clinical responsibilities; these include the fellows and students in rheumatology and especially Steven Abramson, Kathy Haines, Bruce Cronstein, Mark Philips, and Michael Pillinger. Finally, this book would not have been fashioned without the help and instruction of Andrea Cody, whose intelligent attention to a text is a pleasure to acknowledge.

SOURCES

Agassiz, Elizabeth Cary. *Louis Agassiz: His Life and Correspondence.* Boston: Houghton Mifflin, 1886.

Almeida, Hermione de. *Romantic Medicine and John Keats.* Oxford: Oxford University Press, 1991.

Aly, Götz, Peter Chroust, and Christian Pross. *Cleansing the Fatherland: Nazi Medicine and Racial Hygiene.* Baltimore: Johns Hopkins University Press, 1994.

Aptheker, Herbert. *Abolitionism: A Revolutionary Movement.* Boston: Twayne, 1989.

Auden, Wystan Hugh. *Collected Poems.* New York: Vintage, 1991.

Baker, Livia. *The Justice from Beacon Hill: The Life and Times of Oliver Wendell Holmes.* New York: HarperCollins, 1991.

Balderson, Katherine C. "Katharine Lee Bates," in *Notable American Women,* ed. E. T. James. Cambridge: Harvard University Press, 1971.

Ball, George V. "Two Epidemics of Gout," *Bulletin of the History of Medicine,* Vol. 45 (1971), pp. 401–8.

Barlow, Robert B., Dowling, John E., and Weissmann, Gerald, eds. *The Biological Century.* Cambridge: Harvard University Press.

Barzun, Jacques. *A Stroll with William James.* Chicago: University of Chicago Press, 1983.

Bates, Katharine Lee. *Selected Poems.* Boston: Houghton Mifflin, 1930.

Baudelaire, Charles. *Les Fleurs du Mal,* ed. J. Crepet, A. Blin, and C. Pichois. Paris: Gallimard, 1968.

———. *Les Fleurs du Mal,* trans. Richard Howard. Boston: David Godine, 1982.

———. *Oeuvres Complètes,* ed. Y. G. Le Dantec and C. Pichois. Paris: Gallimard, 1961.

Behrman, S. N. *Portrait of Max.* New York: Random House, 1960.

Bell, Joseph. "The Adventures of Sherlock Holmes," *The Bookman*, December 1892, pp. 50–54.

Bell, Millicent. *Meaning in Henry James*. Boston: Harvard University Press, 1991.

Bercovitch, Sacvan. *The Puritan Origins of the American Self.* New Haven: Yale University Press, 1975.

Bernard, Claude. "De l'Origine du Sucre dans l'Economie Animale," *Arch. Gen. Med.*, 4th Series, Vol. 18 (1848), pp. 303–19.

Bichat, Xavier. *Physiological Researches on Life and Death*, trans. F. Gold. London: Longman, 1816.

Blackwell, Elizabeth. *Pioneer Work in Opening the Medical Profession to Women*. London and New York: Longmans, Green, 1895.

Bowen, Catherine Drinker. *Yankee from Olympus: Justice Holmes and His Family*. Boston and New York: Atlantic/Little, Brown, 1944.

Brock, Thomas D. *Robert Koch*. Berlin and New York: Springer Verlag, 1988.

Brooks, Van Wyck. *New England: Indian Summer*. New York: Dutton, 1940.

————. *The Flowering of New England*. New York: Dutton, 1936.

Browne, Thomas. *Religio Medici* (reprint of 1642 with 1678 and 1682 corrections). London: Macmillan, 1881.

Browning, Elizabeth Barrett. *The Letters of Elizabeth Barret Browning*, ed. Frederic G. Kenyon. 2 vols.; London: Macmillan, 1897.

Bruce, George A. *Twentieth Regiment Massachusetts*. Boston: Houghton Mifflin, 1906.

Bryant, William Cullen. *Selected Poems*. New York: Heritage Press, 1947.

Burr, Anna Robeson. *Alice James, Her Brothers, Her Journal.* New York: Dodd, Mead, 1934.

Cannon, Walter B. *The Way of an Investigator*. New York: Norton, 1945.

Capper, Charles. *Margaret Fuller: An American Romantic Life. The Private Years*. New York and Oxford: Oxford University Press, 1992.

Carr, John Dickson. *The Life of Sir Arthur Conan Doyle*. New York: Carroll & Graf, 1987.

Cohen, Alfred E. *Medicine: Science and Art*. Chicago: University of Chicago Press, 1931.

Coleman, William. *Georges Cuvier, Zoologist*. Cambridge: Harvard University Press, 1964.

Conot, R. E. *Justice at Nuremberg*. New York: Carroll & Graf, 1984.

Crane, Sylvia E. *White Silence: Greenough, Powers and Crawford, American Sculptors in Nineteenth-Century Italy.* Coral Gables: University of Miami Press, 1972.

Craven, W. *Sculpture in America.* Newark: University of Delaware Press, 1984.

Cuvier, Georges. *Leçons d'Anatomie Comparée.* 8 vols.; Paris: Crochard, 1800.

———. *The Animal Kingdom*, trans. H. M. McMurtry. 3 vols.; New York: G. & C. H. Carvill, 1831.

Darnton, Robert. *The Great Cat Massacre.* New York: Basic Books, 1984.

———. *Mesmerism and the End of the Enlightenment in France.* Cambridge: Harvard University Press, 1968.

Delbanco, A. *The Puritan Ordeal.* Cambridge: Harvard University Press, 1989.

Dickinson, Emily. *The Poems of Emily Dickinson.* Boston: Harvard University Press, 1951.

Dreyer, W. J., and J. Claude Bennett. "The Molecular Basis of Antibody Formation: A Paradox," *Proceedings of the National Academy of Sciences, USA*, Vol. 54, No. 3 (1965), pp. 864–69.

Duffy, John. *The Sanitarians.* Urbana: University of Illinois Press, 1990.

———. *A History of Public Health in New York, 1866–1966.* New York: Russell Sage Foundation, 1974.

Eliot, George. *Middlemarch.* Boston: Houghton Mifflin, 1956; orig. pub. 1872.

———. *Letters*, ed. G. S. Haight. 12 vols.; New Haven: Yale University Press, 1955.

Emerson, Edwin, Jr. *A History of the Nineteenth Century.* New York: Yale University Press, 1900.

———. *The Life and Letters of Charles Russell Lowell.* Port Washington, N.Y.: Kennikat, 1970; orig. pub. 1907.

Emerson, Ralph Waldo. *The Complete Works.* 6 vols.; Boston: Houghton Mifflin, 1918.

Evans, Richard J. "Cholera in 19th Century Europe," in *Epidemics and Ideas*, ed. T. Ranger and P. Slack. Cambridge: Cambridge University Press, 1992.

Feuer, Lewis S. *The Basic Writings of Marx and Engels.* New York: Doubleday/Anchor, 1959.

Flaubert, Gustave. *Madame Bovary.* New York: Penguin Classics, 1984.

Fleck, Ludwig. *The Genesis and Development of a Scientific Fact.* Chicago: University of Chicago Press, 1979.

Flexner, Abraham. *Medical Education in the United States.* New York: Salem, 1972; orig. pub. 1910.

Flexner, Simon, and James Thomas Flexner. *William Henry Welch and the Heroic Age of American Medicine.* New York: Viking, 1941.

Ford, Worthington Chauncey. *A Cycle of Adams Letters, 1861–1865.* Boston: Houghton Mifflin, 1920.

Forten, Charlotte L. *The Journal of Charlotte L. Forten,* ed. Ray Allen Billington. New York: Norton, 1981.

Foucault, Michel. *The Birth of the Clinic: An Archeology of Medical Perception,* trans. A. M. S. Smith. New York: Random House, 1973.

———. *The Order of Things,* trans. A. M. S. Smith. London: Tavistock, 1970.

Fuller, Margaret. *The Love Letters of Margaret Fuller,* ed. Julia Ward Howe. New York: D. Appleton, 1903.

———. *Woman in the Nineteenth Century and Related Writings.* Boston: J. P. Jewett, 1895.

Garrod, Alfred Baring. *The Nature and Treatment of Gout and Rheumatic Gout.* London: Walton and Maberly, 1859.

Garrod, Archibald Edward. *Inborn Errors of Metabolism.* London: H. Frowde, 1909.

Gooding, Cpl. James Henry. *On the Altar of Freedom: A Black Soldier's Civil War Letters from the Front,* ed. V. M. Adams. Amherst: University of Massachusetts Press, 1991.

Gould, Stephen Jay. *An Urchin in the Storm.* New York: W. W. Norton, 1987.

Grant, Ulysses S. *Memoirs and Selected Letters.* New York: Library of America, 1990.

Habegger, Alfred. *The Father: A Life of Henry James, Sr.* New York: Farrar, Straus & Giroux, 1994.

Hallowell, Norwood Penrose. *The Negro as a Soldier in the War of the Rebellion.* Boston: Little, Brown, 1897.

Hammond, William A. *A Treatise on Diseases of the Nervous System.* New York: D. Appleton, 1871.

———. *A Treatise on Insanity in Its Medical Relation.* New York: D. Appleton, 1883.

Hawthorne, Nathaniel. *The Blithedale Romance.* Columbus: Ohio University Press Centenary Edition, 1964.

———. *The Marble Faun.* Columbus: Ohio University Press Centenary Edition, 1968.

Higginson, Mary Thatcher, ed. *Letters and Journals of Thomas Wentworth Higginson, 1846–1906.* Boston: Houghton Mifflin, 1921.

Higginson, Thomas Wentworth. *Part of a Man's Life.* Port Washington, N.Y.: Kennikat, 1971; orig. pub. 1905.

———. *Army Life in a Black Regiment.* Williamstown, Mass.: Corner House, 1984; orig. pub. 1870.

———. *Margaret Fuller Ossoli.* New York: Chelsea House, 1981; orig. pub. 1857.

Hollander, John. *American Poetry.* 2 vols.; New York: Library of America, 1993.

Holmes, Oliver Wendell. *Collected Works.* 13 vols.; Boston: Houghton Mifflin, 1892.

———. "The Contagiousness of Puerperal Fever," *New England Quarterly Journal of Medicine & Surgery*, Vol. 1 (1842), pp. 503–30.

Howe, Julia Ward. *Reminiscences, 1819–1899.* Boston: Houghton Mifflin, 1899.

James, Henry. *William Wetmore Story and His Friends.* New York: Kennedy/Da Capo, 1961.

James, William. *Essays on Faith, Ethics and Morals.* New York: New American Library, 1974.

———. *Psychology.* 2 vols.; New York: Henry Holt, 1890.

———. *The Will to Believe.* New York: Longmans, Green, 1908.

———. *The Letters of William James*, ed. H. James. Boston: Atlantic Monthly Press, 1920.

Keats, John. *Poetry and Letters*, ed. Elizabeth Cook. New York and Oxford: Oxford University Press, 1990.

Keller, Evelyn Fox. *Feeling for the Organism: The Life and Work of Barbara McClintock.* New York: Freeman, 1983.

———. *Reflections on Gender and Science.* New Haven: Yale University Press, 1992.

Koch, Robert. "Über die Cholerabakterien," *Deutsche Medizinische Wochenschrift*, Vol. 10 (1884), pp. 725–28.

Kruif, Paul de. *Microbe Hunters.* New York: Harcourt, Brace, 1926.

———. *The Sweeping Wind.* New York: Harcourt, Brace & World, 1962.

Larkin, Philip. *Required Writing.* New York: Farrar, Straus & Giroux, 1991.

Leder, Lawrence. *The Bold Brahmins: New England's War Against Slavery, 1831–1863.* New York: Dutton, 1961.

Lewis, Sinclair. *Arrowsmith.* New York: Harcourt, Brace, 1925.

Locke, David. *Science as Writing.* New Haven: Yale University Press, 1992.

Loeb, Jacques. *The Organism as a Whole.* New York: G. Putnam's Sons, 1916.

Lovejoy, Arthur O. *The Great Chain of Being: A Study of the History of an Idea.* Cambridge: Harvard University Press, 1936.

Lowell, James Russell. *Collected Prose Works.* 6 vols.; Boston and New York: Houghton Mifflin, 1892.

———. *Complete Poetical Works.* Boston: Houghton Mifflin, 1897.

Matossian, Mary Kilbourne. *Poisons of the Past: Molds, Epidemics and History.* New Haven: Yale University Press, 1989.

Matthiessen, F. O. *The James Family.* New York: Houghton Mifflin, 1947.

Medawar, Peter. *Pluto's Republic.* Oxford: Oxford University Press, 1982.

Mekalanos, John J., and Jerald C. Sadoff. "Cholera Vaccines: Fighting an Ancient Scourge," *Science,* Vol. 265 (1994), pp. 1387–89.

Monod, Jacques, Jean-Pierre Changeux, and François Jacob. "Allosteric Proteins and Cellular Control Systems," *Journal of Molecular Biology,* Vol. 12 (1963), pp. 88–118.

Morison, Samuel Eliot. *Admiral of the Ocean Sea.* Boston: Little, Brown, 1942.

Morse, John T., Jr. *Oliver Wendell Holmes: Life and Letters.* Boston: Houghton Mifflin, 1893.

Moyers, Bill. *Healing and the Mind.* New York: Doubleday, 1993.

Norton, Charles Eliot, ed. *The Letters of James Russell Lowell.* New York: Harper & Bros., 1904.

———. *Correspondence Between Thomas Carlyle and Ralph Waldo Emerson.* Boston: James R. Osgood, 1883.

Novick, Sheldon M. *Honorable Justice: The Life of Oliver Wendell Holmes.* Boston and New York: Little, Brown, 1989.

Oates, Stephen B. *To Purge This Land of Blood: A Biography of John Brown.* Amherst: University of Massachusetts Press, 1984.

Palmer, George Herbert. *The Life of Alice Freeman Palmer.* Boston: Houghton Mifflin, 1908.

Perry, Bliss. *The Heart of Emerson's Journals.* Boston: Houghton Mifflin, 1926.

Poe, Edgar Allan. *The Complete Poems and Stories with Selected Critical Writings.* New York: Knopf, 1946.

Richards, Iawa E. *Letters and Journal of Samuel Gridley Howe.* 2 vols.; Boston: Dana Estes, 1909.

Rose, Phyllis. *Parallel Lives*. New York: Vintage, 1983.

Rosenberg, Charles. *The Cholera Years*. Chicago: University of Chicago Press, 1962.

Rothfield, Lawrence. *Vital Signs*. Princeton: Princeton University Press, 1992.

Schama, Simon. *Dead Certainties*. New York: Knopf, 1991.

Scudder, Vida. *On Journey*. Boston: Houghton Mifflin, 1937.

Seigel, J. *Bohemian Paris*. New York: Elisabeth Sifton Books, 1986.

Semmelweis, Ignaz Philipp. *Die Ätiologie, der Begriff und die Prophylaxis des Kindbettfiebers Pest*. Vienna and Leipzig: C. A. Hartleben, 1861.

Serventi, I. M., and J. Moss. "Enhancement of Cholera Toxin-Catalyzed ADP-Ribosylation by Guanine Nucleotide-Binding Proteins," *Current Topics in Microbiology and Immunology*, Vol. 175 (1992), pp. 43–67.

Shaw, Robert Gould. *"Blue-Eyed Child of Fortune": The Civil War Letters of Colonel Robert Gould Shaw*, ed. Russell Duncan. Athens: University of Georgia Press, 1992.

Sherman, William Tecumseh. *Memoirs*. New York: Library of America, 1990.

Shorter, Edward. *From Paralysis to Fatigue: A History of Psychosomatic Illness in the Modern Era*. New York: Free Press, 1992.

Silverman, Kenneth. *Edgar A. Poe*. New York: Harper Perennial, 1991.

Snow, Charles P. *The Two Cultures and the Scientific Revolution*. Cambridge: Cambridge University Press, 1959.

Snow, John. "On the Pathology and Mode of Communication of the Cholera," *London Medical Gazette*, Vol. 44 (1849), pp. 730–32, 745–52, 923–29.

Solomons, L. M., and G. Stein. "Normal Motor Automatism," *Psychological Review*, Vol. 2 (1896), pp. 492–512.

Stendhal [Henri Beyle]. *The Life of Henri Brulard*. New York: Vintage, 1955.

Strouse, Jean. *Alice James*. Boston: Houghton Mifflin, 1980.

Szent-Györgyi, Albert. *The Crazy Ape*. New York: Philosophical Library, 1970.

Taylor, Robert. *Saranac: America's Magic Mountain*. Boston: Houghton Mifflin, 1986.

Thomas, Lewis. *Lives of a Cell: Notes of a Biology Watcher*. New York: Viking, 1977.

——. *The Youngest Science: Notes of a Medicine Watcher*. New York: Viking, 1983.

————. "Adaptive Aspects of Inflammation," in *Immunology of Inflammation*, ed. B. K. Forscher and J. C. Houck. Amsterdam: Excerpta Medica, 1971.

Thomas, Robert Davis. *With Bleeding Footsteps: Mary Baker Eddy's Path to Religious Leadership*. New York: Knopf, 1994.

Thomson, Elizabeth H. "Elizabeth Blackwell," in *Notable American Women*, ed. E. T. James. Cambridge: Harvard University Press, 1971.

Tilton, Eleanor M. *Amiable Autocrat: A Biography of Dr. Oliver Wendell Holmes*. New York: Henry Schuman, 1947.

Tocqueville, Alexis de. *Recollections*. New York: Doubleday, 1970.

Trilling, Lionel. *The Liberal Imagination*. New York: Doubleday/Anchor, 1950.

————. *Sincerity and Authenticity*. Cambridge: Harvard University Press, 1971.

Wade, Mason. *Margaret Fuller: Whetstone of Genius*. New York: Viking, 1940.

Ward, Aileen. *John Keats: The Making of a Poet*. New York: Viking, 1963.

Watson, James. *The Double Helix*. New York: Atheneum, 1968.

———— and Francis H. C. Crick. "Molecular Structure of Nucleic Acids: A Structure for Deoxyribose Nucleic Acid," *Nature*, Vol. 171 (1953), pp. 737–38.

Wayman, Dorothy A. *Edward Sylvester Morse*. Cambridge: Harvard University Press.

Weissmann, Gerald, ed. *The Biological Revolution: Applications of Cell Biology to Public Welfare*. New York: Plenum Press, 1979.

Weissmann, Gerald, ed. "Advances in Inflammation Research," Vol. 1 (1979), pp. 1–64.

————. *Mediators of Inflammation*. New York: Plenum, 1974.

———— and Lewis Thomas. "Studies on Lysosomes. I. The Effects of Endotoxin. Endotoxin Tolerance and Cortisone on Release of Acid. Hydrolases from a Granular Fraction of Rabbit Liver," *Journal of Experimental Medicine*, Vol. 116 (1962), pp. 451–66.

Williams, William Carlos. *Selected Poems*. New York: New Directions, 1949.

Wilson, Edmund. *The Forties*, ed. Leon Edel. New York: Farrar, Straus & Giroux, 1983.

————. *Patriotic Gore*. Oxford and New York: Oxford University Press, 1962.

————. *The Sixties*, ed. Leon Edel. New York: Farrar, Straus & Giroux, 1993.

INDEX